IMMUNE SYSTEM
AND
CHINESE HERBS

by

Pi-Kwang Tsung, Ph.D.

1989

INSTITUTE OF CHINESE HERB

ISBN: 0-613-19320-1

Published by the Institute of Chinese Herb
16 Almond Tree Lane, Irvine, California 92715
First printing, 1989

Printed in United States of America

ABOUT THE AUTHOR

Dr. Pi-kwang Tsung has a distinguished background in research and teaching, and has broad knowledge in agricultural chemistry, microbiology, biochemistry, pharmaceutical science, and clinical chemistry. He has been awarded the Hu Tieh-hua Scholarship (Taiwan), the Yoneyama Rotary Club Foundation Scholarship (Japan) and the Overseas Trainees Scholarship of Scientists (Japan).

After earning his M.S. degree in agricultural chemistry from Tokyo University, Dr. Tsung studied microbiology at the University of Kansas, where he obtained an M.A. degree with a thesis on Q-fever before returning to Tokyo University to complete his doctorate in pharmaceutical science in 1970. He has since served as a research scientist at the New York University Medical Center; Assistant Professor of pathology at the University of Connecticut Health Center; principal investigator in a research project in muscular dystrophy at St. Elizabeth's Hospital, Boston; and advisor on ocular biochemistry to the Dry Eye Institute in Lubbock, Texas. Past Executive Director of the Oriental Healing Arts Institute, he also was Editor-in-Chief of the Oriental Healing Arts International Bulletin. He is the current President of Institute of Chinese Herb.

Dr. Tsung is the author of more than seventy scientific papers, including numerous studies on leukocyte chemotaxis, protein phosphorylation in control mechanisms, muscular dystrophy, tear film physiology, glaucoma, and retina disease. He is also the author of "Immunology and Chinese Herbal Medicine", "Allergy and Chinese Herbal Medicine", and "Arthritis and the Chinese Herbal Medicine".

Dr. Tsung has been invited by the Chinese Association of the Integration of the Traditional and Western Medicine to give lectures at the China Academy of Traditional Chinese Medicine. He has also been a guest lecturer at Nanjing College of Traditional Chinese Medicine.

ACKNOWLEDGEMENTS

I wish to thank Dr. Keith Borton for information on his Chinese herbal treatment of AIDS patients.

I also wish to thank Mr. W.S. Yang for the financial support.

Pi-Kwang Tsung, Ph.D.
Irvine, California
May, 1989

NOTICE

The therapies discussed in this book are strictly adjunctive or complementary to medical treatment. Self-treatment for a serious ailment can be dangerous. Therefore, you are urged to seek the advice of a Chinese herbal doctor or else the best medical assistance available whenever it is needed.

TABLE OF CONTENTS

Preface

This book has been designed not to bombard the reader with terminology, but rather to explain in simple language updated information on Chinese herbs and the immune system. Medical terminology is defined and the scientific and Chinese name of all herbs mentioned in text are listed in the accompanying glossary and appendixes.

Chinese herbal formula terminology has been very confused by its English names, Chinese pinyin, and Japanese names. In order to let readers know which ones are identical, a table is furnished for this purpose.

Formulas for aging-associated diseases and herbs possessing anti- AIDS virus, interferon-inducing activity, and immunostimulating activity are listed in appendixes. The commonly used marker constituents of Chinese herbs are also listed in appendixes.

A strong effort has been put on the scientific verification of Chinese herb and Chinese herbal formula applications.

I
Introduction

Chinese herbal medicine is still used as a practical medical treatment by hundreds of millions of Chinese and other Orientals. Since it is characteristic of Chinese herbal medicine not only to cure disease but also to restore the normal functions of the body in order to strengthen the patient's resistance, re-evaluation of Chinese herbal medicines could lead to the discovery of new treatments of many diseases. In Japan, Chinese herbal medicine has been adapted to physicians' prescriptions, and Chinese herbal medicine co-exists well with Western medicine in the Japanese medical system. Chinese herbal medicine has become immensely popular in Japan during this decade, and Chinese herbal medicine has also increased in popularity in the United States as people become aware of Western drugs' hazardous side-effects.

Most Chinese herbal medicines, whether they consist of single herbs or combined formulas, are adaptogenic and tonic immunostimulants. They stimulate blood flow or microcirculation, enhance phagocytosis in the reticuloendothelial system, and affect metabolism and the endocrine system. The search for drugs capable of stimulating or modulating our immune systems is worldwide, and comprises activities in a variety of research disciplines. A great many specific immunological in vitro and in vivo test systems, which allow constituents to be selected and screened for potential immunological activities, are available today. The identification of many immunostimulating polysaccharides in anti-cancer Chinese herbs also brings us the potential for fighting cancer by enhancing our own immune systems with the help of these immunostimulating polysaccharides or these immunopolysaccharide-rich Chinese herbs. These immunostimulating polysaccharides are also able to suppress the metastasis of cancer after cancer surgery and are able to relieve the side effects of radiotherapy and chemotherapy in cancer treatment. In addition, interferon-inducing activity, tumor necrosis factor, mitogenic activity for lymphocytes, anti-viral activity including anti-human immunodeficiency virus activity, and factors for clearing circulating immune complexes have been identified from many Chinese herbs which lead to wider use of Chinese herbs to treat AIDS patients in acupuncture clinics and Western medical clinics.

Eternal youth, or an elixir of life, has been an active human quest since ancient times. Many scientists believe that our maximum lifespan is about 110 to 140 years. Unfortunately, our immune functions decrease with age. Cancer, atherosclerosis, hypertension, diabetes, nephrosis, rheumatoid arthritis, and Alzheimer's Disease are typical diseases associated with the aging process. The quest for eternal youth, and a healthy and happy life will be much in demand from now on. Using immunostimulaling Chinese herbs in our daily diets can not only boost our immune system against diseases, but also keep us younger for a happier, healthier life.

II
Immunology in
Chinese Herbal Medicine

A. The Concept of the Immune System

The human body has a defense system which can recognize and eliminate foreign bodies when it is invaded by such bodies.

The human red blood cells have an antigen-recognizing ability which distinguishes their own cell type from others. Therefore, human blood is assigned to blood groups A,B, AB, or O, depending on whether the red cells carry the A antigen, the B antigen, both, or neither of these antigens. Human beings of blood group B will respond to an injection of A red cells by producing anti-A antibodies. They do not produce anti-B antibodies because the B antigen is not foreign to them. The white blood cells, leukocytes, also have the ability to recognize and reject a foreign organ when it is transplanted from one individual to a different individual. This human leukocyte antigen is commonly abbreviated HLA, and is another way in which the parts of the human body distinguish "self" from "non-self."

Since microbes have existed on earth for several billion years longer than human beings and animals have, both human beings and animals need a good defense system in order to survive. The animal body possesses leukocytes and macrophages for the phagocytosis of foreign invaders, and lymphocytes, γ-globulin, and a complemntary system for inactivating invaders. Human leukocytes, macrophages, lymphocytes, and complementary systems can also recognize and eliminate foreign invaders, transformed cells, cell debris and cancer cells. This defense system is called the immune system. When this immune system is functioning normally, we should not feel any symptoms of illness in our bodies. However, when the immunological activity is decreased or too many antigens are overpowering the defense system, then we will feel such symptoms as fever, pain, swelling, or itching until a normal condition is recovered.

The symptoms of the different stages of immunological reactions can be assigned to the defense systems of inflammation and allergy.

B. Immunology in Chinese Herbal Medicine

The concept equivalent to immunology appeared in the ancient and legendary medical classic "The Yellow Emperor's Treatise on Internal Medicine" (Wang, 762 A.D.) traditionally attributed to the early Han dynasty (206 B.C. - 23 A.D.). In its second chapter, simple questions on the great treatise on the harmony of the atmosphere of the four seasons with the spirit clearly purposed that preventive treatment is better than that undertaken after the occurrence of disease. The third-century "Treatise on Febrile Diseases" (Chang, 219 A.D.)contains significant observations on the symptoms of diseases and the practical application of Chinese herbal formulas. Even though the names of diseases described in the "Treatise on Febrile Diseases" are not the same as those ascribed by modern medicine, the careful descriptions and studies of the symptoms are well matched to the modern term "immunology," "inflammation," and "allergy." Both the "Treatise on Febrile Diseases" and "The Yellow Emperor's Treatise on Internal Medicine" postulated that various disease-causing factors (evil elements) are in the environment and outside the human body. The "evil elements" in modern terms are virus, bacteria, fungi, and allergen. The ancient Chinese believed that in the course of the struggle between genuine energy (vitality, resistance) and these evil elements, the firmness or weakness of the genuine energy would directly decide the occurrence, development, processes, and results of diseases.

Scientific evidence that sickness originates from the invasion of microbes was obtained after the invention of the microscope. Edward Jenner introduced vaccination in 1796, but almost a century elapsed before Jenner's vaccine was followed by others when Louis Pasteur ushered in the modern era of immunology. In 1884, Ilia Ilich Metchnikoff found that leukocytes and macrophages are involved in the defense mechanisms of human and animal bodies. The whole concept of the immune system, involving the recognition of "self" and "non-self" and the elimination of foreign agents, was not even suggested before the discovery of vaccination and the phagocytic function of leucocytes and macrophages.

It is quite surprising, therefore, that the ancient Chinese postulated the antigen (evil element) and anticipated immune- system theory by prescribing herb combinations for this purpose.

C. Immunologically Active Polysaccharides Isolated
   from Chinese Herbs

The components of Chinese herbs play an important role in promoting homeostasis in the body's biological system. Recently, Polysaccharide fractions from Chinese herbal medicine have been shown to have interferon-inducing activity, anti-tumor activity, mitogenic activity for lymphocytes, stimulating activity for phagocytic function of the reticuloendothelial system, and anti-inflammatory activity; they also act as immunosuppressants and stimulate the production of antibodies. The low-molecular-weight components in Chinese herbs have been studied in detail. However, the high-molecular-weight polysaccharide components have not received much attention until recent years. Since the finding of anti-tumor activity in polysaccharide fractions from Chinese herbs, investigation of the structure and pharmacology of these polysaccharides has been intensified in many countries, especially in Japan. Table 1 lists Chinese herbs which have been used in cancer therapy in China for many years. The active components have been identified as polysaccharides.

The chemical properties of anti-tumor polysaccharides found in Chinese herbs are listed in Table 2.

All the immunologically active polysaccharides have been found to contain $\beta(1\rightarrow3)$ glucan as the main chain linkage in their structures. Further investigation revealed that none of the polysaccharides were either mutagenic or carcinogenic. Polysaccharides may therefore be promising agents for future immunostimulatory medications.

The research group in the Oriental Medicine Research Center of the Kitasato Institute in Japan has further identified immunomodulating arabinogalactan in Chinese herbs. Table 3 shows the water-soluble immunomodulating arabinogalactan and arabinogalactan containing polysaccharides from Chinese herbs. All of the isolated polysaccharides have an arabinogalactan portion with an arabino-3.6-galactan structure. Recently, a water-soluble polysaccharide isolated from panax notoginseng was shown to have a stimulatory effect on the phagocytic activity of reticuloendothelial systems. The water-soluble polysaccharide of panax notoginseng is also an arabino-3.6-galactan with arabinofuranose as the terminal sugar (Ohtani, et al, 1985). The results strongly suggest that the polysaccharides in the Chinese medicines play an important role in modulation of immune function.

Table 1. Anticancer Chinese herbs and their major actions

Herbs	Active components	Major actions
Astragalus mongholicus (leguminosae)	Polysaccharides	intensifies phagocytosis of reticuloendothelial systems and the pituitary-adrenal cortical function; restores hematopoetic function of bone marrow
Codonopsis tangshen (Campanulaceae)	saponins polysaccharides	enhances phagocytosis of macrophagocytes; counteracts leukopenia induced by chemotherapy or radiotherapy
Panax ginseng (Araliaceae)	ginsenosides panaxosides panaxatriol	enhances pituitary-adrenal cortical functionand phagocytic activity of macrophagocytes; increases content of immunoglobulin and cAMP in the adrenal gland; promotes lymphocytic transformation; restores hematopoietic fumction of bome marrow; increases hemoglobulin
Eleutherococcus senticosis (Araliaceae)	eleutherosides polysaccharides	possesses actions similar to those of Panax ginseng; counteracts x-ray radiation, leukemia, and drug-induced tumors; inhibits metastasis
Poria cocos (Polyporaceae)	polysaccharides pachymaran	restores antitumor immuno-surveillant system
Lentinus edodes (Polyporaceae)	polysaccharides	possesses actions similar to those of ling-chih
Glycyrrhiza echinata (Leguminosae)	glycyrrhizin	intensifies pituitary-adrenal cortical function; inhibits cAMP phosphatase and increases content of cAMP in cardiac and pyloric mucus memberane; inhibits gastric tumors
Ganoderma lucidum (polyporaceae)	polysaccharides	increases level of cellular immunity; inhibits growth of tumor cells
Oldenlandia diffusa (Rubiaceae)		stimulates reticuloendothelial system; intensifies phagocytosis
Polyporus umbellatus (Polyporaceae)	polysaccharides Gu-1	regulates and stimulates immune system; promotes transformation of cancer cells into mormal cells

(From Nanking Pharmacy College, 1976; Chendu Traditional Medical College, 1978; Tao, 1981)

Table 2. Structures of Anti-Tumor Polysaccharides Found in Chinese Herbs.

Herb	Polysaccharides	Linkage		References
		Main Chain	Side Chain	
Cordyceps ophio - glossoides	CO-1	$\beta(1\rightarrow3)G$	$\beta(1\rightarrow6)g$	Yamada et al.(1984)
Coriolus versicolor	Klestin(PSK)	$\beta(1\rightarrow4)G$ $\beta(1\rightarrow6)G$	$\beta(1\rightarrow6)g$	Hirase et al.(1976)
Ganoderma lucidum	GL-1	$\beta(1\rightarrow3)G$	$\alpha(1\rightarrow4)G$ $\beta(1\rightarrow6)G$ $\beta(1\rightarrow3)G$	Miyazaki et al.(1981) Ukai et al.(1982)
	GA-1	$\beta(1\rightarrow3)G$	$\beta(1\rightarrow6)G$	
Lentinus edodes	lentinan	$\beta(1\rightarrow3)G$	$\beta(1\rightarrow6)G$	Sasaki et al.(1976)
Omphalia lapidescens, Polyporus mylittae	OL-2	$\beta(1\rightarrow3)G$	$\beta(1\rightarrow6)G$	Miyazaki et al. (1981)
Polyporus umbellatus	GU-2	$\beta(1\rightarrow6)G$ $\beta(1\rightarrow3)G$	$\beta(1\rightarrow6)G$ $\alpha(1\rightarrow4)G$	Miyazaki et al. (1978,1979)
	GU-3	$\beta(1\rightarrow3)G$	$\beta(1\rightarrow6)G$ $\alpha(1\rightarrow4)G$	Miyazaki et al. (1978,1979)
	GU-4	$\beta(1\rightarrow3)G$		"　　　"
	AP	$\beta(1\rightarrow3)G$	$\beta(1\rightarrow6)G$	Ueno et al.(1982)
Poria cocos	pachymaram	$\beta(1\rightarrow3)G$		Chihara (1978)

G = glucose

Table 3. Water-soluble immunomodulating arabinogalactan containing polysaccharides from Chinese herbs

Herb	Polysaccharides	Sugar content (mole ratio)	Type of arabinogalactan	Pharmacological activity	Reference
Artemisia argyi	AAFIb-2	Rha:Xyl:Ara:Gal:Glc:UroA (2.5:2.5:4:3.6:1.0:59.4%)	II	Anti-complementary activity	Yamada et al, (1985a,1985b,1985c)
	AFIIb-3	Rha:Xyl:Ara:Gal:Glc:UroA (1.5:1.0:9.4:7.5:1.0:49%)	II	Anti-complementary activity	Yamada et al, (1985a,1985b,1985c)
Coix lachrymajobi	CA-1	Rha:Ara:Xyl:Gal:Glc:UroA (1.8:43.8:10.8:33.2:trace:10.4)	II	Anti-complementary activity	Yamada et al., (1985a)
	CA-2	Rha:Ara:Xyl:Man:Gal:Glc:UroA (2.4:37.0:11.8:1.7:35.6:2.9:8.6)	II	Anti-complementary activity	Yamada et al, (1985a)
Lithospermum euchromum	LR-IIa	Rha:Fue:Ara:Xyl:Man:Gal:Glc:UroA (2.0:2.5:3.4:2.8:5.6:9.6:14.4:15%)	II	Anti-complementary activity	Yamada et al, (in press)
Panax notoginseng	2A-AG	Ara:Gal:Glc(23:75:2)	II	Stimulation of RES phagocytic activity	Ohtani et al, (1985)
Angelica acutiloba	AGIIa	Ara:Gal(1.2:1.0)	II	Anti-complementary activity	Yamada et al, (1985d)
	AGIIb-1	Ara:Gal:Rha:UroA(2.2:1.0:0.3:0.5)	II	Anti-complementary activity	Kiyohara et al, (1985 a,b)

Ara = arabinose, Gal = galactose, Rha = rhamnose, UroA = uronic acid
Xyl = xylose, Man = Mannose, Fuc = fucose, Glc = glucose

It has been shown that the active site and inhibitory site of anti-complementary polysaccharide are co-existing in the polysaccharide structure (Kiyohara, et al, 1985; Nagai, et al, 1985). Therefore, it can be assumed that the pharmacological effect of Chinese herbal medicine is regulated in the Yin-Yang way.

III
Anti-Cancer and
Immunostimulating
Polysaccharides

A. Introduction

Studies of biologically or immunologically active polysaccharides can be said to constitute the history of the search for anti- cancer agents from an immunotherapeutical viewpoint.

In China and Japan, the Chinese herbs ginseng, hoelen, codonopsis, polyporus, astragalus, ganoderma, ficus, dandelion, lentinus, brasenia, aloe, and laminaria, all of which have a high polysaccharide content, have been used as anti-cancer medications (see Table 4).

In Europe, Lewisohn's group in 1941 observed that the continued administration of a polysaccharide fraction extracted from bread yeasts could cure 30% of breast cancer of A/J mice. This report was confirmed by Snell of the Jackson Laboratory. About 15 years after Lewisohn's discovery, Diller's group (1963) and Stock's group (Bradner et al, 1958; 1959) used yeast cell walled zymosan and hydroglucan to cure transplanted cancers such as Sarcoma-180 and Sarcoma-37 in Swiss mice. They reported that the anti-cancer effect of zymosan or hydroglucan was due to a host mediated antitumor mechanism rather than a direct cytotoxic effect.

Table 4. Anti-Cancer Chinese Herbs with High Polysaccharide Content

Common name	Botanical name
Aloe	Aloe vera L.
Astragalus	Astragalus hoantchy Franchet
Brasenia	Brasenia schreberi Gmel
Codonopsis	Codonopsis tangshen Oliv
Dandelion	Taraxicum mongolicum Hand-Mazz
Ficus	Ficus carica L.
Ganoderma	Ganoderma lucidum (Leyss. ex Fr.)
Ginseng	Panax ginseng Meyer
Hoelen	Poria cocos(Schw.) Walf
Laminaria	Laminaria japonica Aresch.
Lentinus	Lentinus edodes (Berk.) Sing.
Polyporus	Polyporus umbellatus (Pers.) Fr.

Because Diller and Stock's reports were so sensational at that time, most researchers believed that the anti-cancer effect of polysaccharide was not specific to cancer cells but due to the enhancement effect of graft versus host reaction. It was considered a similar phenomenon as to the enhancement effect of the rejection reaction by the body when an individual was transplanted with a heart or kidney. However, the effect was not understood by the researchers at that time, because the late 1950s was only the beginning of the modern cellular immunology and immunogenetics era.

Since the establishment of genetically syngeneic animals by the Jackson Laboratory and cancer immunology by Gross (1943), Foley (1953), and Prehn (1957), using immunostimulants against cancer has become an exciting topic among cancer researchers. In these two decades, the rapid development of cellular immunology and cancer immunology has brought us hope to control the immune response and suppress cancer growth. The anti-cancer and immunostimulating effects of ploysaccharides should be taken into consideration as the anti-aging substance since our immunities is decrease with age.

B . Anti-Cancer Polysaccharides: Structure-Activity Relationship

The most studied polysaccharides for clinic or drug development for anti-cancer and immuno-stimulant are glucans and mannans, especially lentinan from Lentinus edodes and DL-yeast glucan.

Anti-cancer and immunological activities of the polysaccharides depend not only on the primary structure but also on their conformation and micelles structure. As shown in Table 5, β-(1→3) the main chain of the polysaccharide has demonstrated strong activity against Sarcoma-180. This includes lentinan, schizophyllan and pachymaran. However, structures such as pachyman and laminaran showed no activity at all. Pusturan (GE-3) has strong anti-cancer activity with the β-(1→6) structure in the main chain of the polysaccharide. However, pachyman also has the β-(1→6) structure in the main chain but still no acitivity. When pachyman was treated with 4 molar urea at 45°C for 4 hours a strong anti-cancer activity was shown. This shows that the conformation of the polysaccharide also plays an important role for the anti-cancer activity.

The anti-tumor polysaccharides found in Chinese herbs also show β-(1→3) and β-(1→6) linkage in the polysaccharide structure (Table 5).

Table 5. Polysaccharide Structure and Anti-Cancer (Sarcoma-180) Effect.

Polysaccharides	Primary Structure	Activity against Sarcoma-180	
		Dosage(mg/kg/day)	Inhibitory Effect(%)
Lentinan	β-(1→6)(1→3)-G	1x10	100
Pachyman	β-(1→6)(1→3)-G	5x10	0
Urea-treated pachyman	β-(1→6)(1→3)-G	5x10	91.4
Hydroxyethyl pachyman	β-(1→6)(1→3)-G	5x10	100
Schizophyllan	β-(1→6)(1→3)-G	1x10	100
Scleroglucan	β-(1→6)(1→3)-G	3x10	89.3
Straight chain lentinan	β-(1→3)-G	2x5	90.0
Laminaran	β-(1→3)-G	25x10	1.5
Pachymaran	β-(1→3)-G(straight chain)	5x10	88.0
Pusturan(GE-3)[a]	β-(1→6)-G	200x10	99.1
LC-12[b]	α-(1→6)-G	5x10	-17.6
Dextran	α-(1→6)-G	10x10	-21.2
CM-cellulose[c]	β-(1→4)-G	10x10	4.5
AR[d]	β-(1→2)-G	5x10	0
DL-yeast glucan	β-(1→6)(1→3)-G		+ +
Levan	β-(2→6) furactan		+ +
Klestin	β-(1→4)-β-(1→3)β-(1→6)-G	1000x20	75.9

a) Polysaccharide from parmelia Saxalilis Ach
b) Polysaccharide from Lentinus edodes
c) CM-cellulose: Carboxylethyl cellulose
d) Polysaccharide from Agronobacterium radiogenesis
G = glucan
(Chihara, G, 1981)

C. Immunostimulating Polysaccharides from Ginseng

Ginseng has been claimed to increase resistance to disease, renew vitality for the aging, have natural stimulation of the system, and have an adaptogenic function.

Immunostimulating polysaccharide isolated from Panax ginseng enhances petuitary-adrenal cortical function and phagocytic activity of phagocytes. The polysaccharide also increases content of immunoglobulin and cyclic AMP in the adrenal gland. It promotes lymphocytic transformation and restores hematopoietic function of bone marrow (Tao, et al, 1981). Eleuterococcus senticosis, the common name as siberian ginseng, also possesses activities similar to those of panax ginseng. Immunostimulating polysaccharede from panax notoginseng stimulates phagocytic activity of reticuloendothelial system (Ohtani et al, 1985). Most anti-cancer polysaccharides are also immunostimulants.

D. The Functional Mechanism of Anti-Cancer and immunostimulating Polysaccharides

There are many suggestions concerning the anti-cancer and immunostimulating mechanisms of polysaccharides. The functions of the polysaccharides include intensified phagocytosis of reticuloendotherlial systems, activation of macrophages, activation of T-lymphocytes, enhancement of cell-mediated immune response, and activation of the alternative pathway of the complement system.

The polysaccharide lentinan isolated from the Chinese herb Hsiang-ku (Lentinus edodes) has been mostly studied for its effects on immunostimulation and anti-cancer action. Therefore, an anti-cancer and immunostimulating mechanism of lentinan is shown in Fig. 1. One of the mechanisms is non-specifically induced cytotoxic macrophage which attacks and destroyes cancer cells through the activation of the third complement, C3. In this mechanism, lentinan activates the complement system and increases C3, then C3 is hydrolyzed to C3a and C3b (Okuda et al, 1972; Hamuro et al, 1978). C3a acts directly to destroy cancer cells. However, C3b activates macrophages inducing lysosomal enzymes production and non-specifically destroyes target cancer cells (Hamuro et al, 1980).

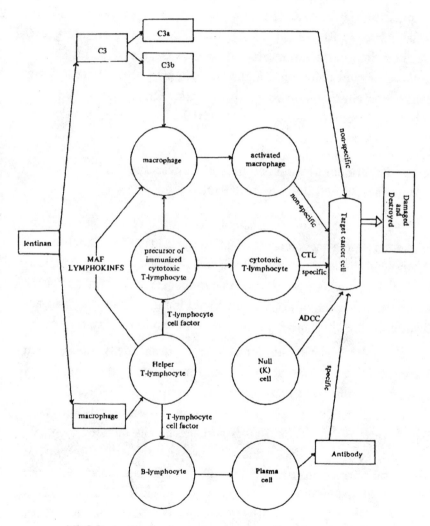

ADCC: Antibody-dependent cell-mediated cytotoxicity

Figure 1. Anti-cancer and immunostimulating mechanism of lentinan.

The second mechanism of immunoactivation and anti-cancer action of lentinan is to kill cancer cells through activation of T- lymphocytes. Lentinan loses its anti-cancer activity in thymusectomy mice (Maeda and Chihara, 1971). However, T lymphocytes are not the only cells contributing to anti-cancer activity. First, lentinan has to activate marcophages for production of lymphocyte activating factor (LAF). Then LAF stimulates helper T-lymphocyte to release different kinds of helper T-lymphocyte factors (Akigama and Hamuro, 1981). The helper T-lymphocyte factor is one kind of lymphokines. One of the factors is called interleukin-2 which is believed to play an important role in converting immature cytotoxic T-lymphocyte. Only mature cytotoxic T-lymphocytes can kill cancer cells.

In another route, T-lymphocyte factors stimulate to become plasma cells to produce humoral antibody and cooperate with null (killer) cells to kill target cancer cells specifically by antibody-dependent cell-mediated cytotoxicity. Macrophage activating factor, one of the helper T-lymphocyte factors, also plays an important role in antibody-dependent macrophage-mediated cytotoxicity for the cancer cell killing mechanism. Lentinan- induced helper T-lymphocyte factor is also involved in the release of natural killer cell activating factor in virus-induced cancer.

In most of the cancer-host relationships, cancer destruction is accomplished by many different routes. Which route will be the major function depends on the cancer-host relationship, genetic factors, and the amount and strength of the antigen. In general, when macrophages are active then the activity of lymphocytes are low. In other words, when lymphocytes are active then the macrophage activity is low. Similarily, when humoral immune response is activated then the cellular immunity is weaker. The opposite is also true. The biological system is always maintained in balance for good health.

E. Immunostimulating Polysaccharides as a Preventive
   Medicine or Health Food

Our immunities decrease with age. The decrease of immunities can result in contracting many diseases, such as cancer, diabetes, arthritis, nephrosis and infection. Since immunostimulating polysaccharides can stimulate our immune system, the polysaccharides can be considered as a preventive medicine or health food. They might be helpful in the management of Acquired Immune Deficiency Syndrome (AIDS) since the main function of the polysaccharides is the stimulation of immune responses.

F. Clinical Application of the Immunostimulating
   Polysaccharides for Cancer Treatment

It has been shown that the immunostimulating polysaccharedes have no toxic effect on humans (Taguchi,1980). The application of the polysaccharides in the clinic is safe as shown by animal and human tests (Taguchi, 1980). However, the timing of the administration, schedule of the administration and combined use with other therapy and surgery need to be studied in detail in order to know more about the cancer cell-host relationship. Multiplicity and diversity of cancer also cause difficulties in cancer therapy. Immunostinulating polysaccharides alone for cancer treatment have been reviewed by many researchers. Therefore, this section will not discuss this matter. The following are the clinical applications that can be expected to be successful.

(A) Administration of the polysaccharide before surgery can suppress the metastasis of cancer

The control of metastasis is a problem in cancer. The control of metastasis after surgery is a key for successful surgery.

Whole cells or cell walls of Bacillus of Calmette and Guerin (BCG)(Zbar et al, 1972; Bansal and Sjogren, 1973; Sparks et al, 1973, 1974; Smith et al, 1976) and Corynebacterium parvum (Milas and Mujagic, 1972; Pol-Deprum and Chouroulinkov, 1973;Bomford and Olivotto, 1974; Bomford et al,1975) have been found to be effective in preventing the metastasis of cancer after surgery. Theoretically, the immunostimulating effect of bacterial whole cells, bacterial cell walls and purified immunostimualting polysaccharides are similar except purified immunostimualting polysaccharides do not contain pyrogen, which causes high fever. The disadvantage of using whole cells and cell walls is that pyrogens are in the preparation. Therefore, purified immunostimulating polysaccharides are more suitable for clinical application.

(B) Combined use of anti-cancer or immunostimulating polysaccharides with radiation therapy in cancer patients

Ginseng extract has been found to have a radiation protection effect (Yonezawa et al, 1981, 1985). The radiation protective principle is not ginseng saponin (Yonezawa et al, 1981). It has been demonstrated that polysaccharides from yeast can induce radiation protection and significantly decrease the mortality of mice exposed to X-rays (Maisin et al, 1986). The radiation protection principle of ginseng extract is suggested to be polysaccharide in nature (Yonezawa et al, 1987). Immunostimulating Chinese herbs also have radiaton protection activity (Yonezawa et al, 1987). The combined use of immunostimulating polysaccharide with radiation therapy for cancer treatment will be very beneficial to cancer patients.

(C) Combined use of anti-cancer or immunostinulating polysaccharides with chemotherapy in cancer patients

It seems to be contradictory in principle to combine an immunostimulating polysaccharide with an immunosuppresive drug for cancer therapy. However, diversity of the functional mechanism of immunostimulating polysaccharides (Tsung and Hsu, 1986) and multiplicity of cancer states with the diversity of immunosuppressive mechanism in cancer allow the immunostimulant and immunosuppressor to act on different cells and different sites. Chinese herbal medicines have been formulated this way for more than 2,000 years and it works in the Yin-Yang way.

Combination of BCG and cyclophosphamide or BCNU (1,3-bis (2- chloroethyl)-1-nitrosourea) have been successful in treating leukemia and lymphoma(Pearson et al, 1972, 1973, 1974, 1975; Sher et al, 1973). The combination of Corynebacterum parvum and cyclophosphamide also succeeded in treating chemical-induced cancer in mice (Currie and Bagshawe, 1970). Immumostimulating polysaccharides should be as successful in combination with chemotherapy as BCG and Corynebacteria.

G. Tumor Necrosis Factor-producing Chinese Herbs

Tumor necrosis factor (TNF) was first described by Carswell et al (1975) as a factor in serum obtained from mice, rats, or rabbits which caused regression of some transplanted tumor cells in vivo and was cytostatic or cytocidal to some tumor cells in culture. TNF is an active component of antitumor activity. Highly active TNF activity can be obtained with the extract of Chinese herbs such as angelica root, bupleurum root, cnidium rhizome, or cinnamon bark (Haranaka, Satomi, et al, 1985). The antitumor activities and capacity for TNF production of the Chinese herbal extracts are probably due partly to stimulation of the reticuloendothelial system and the induction of host-mediated antitumor substances like TNF.

H. Concluding Remarks

To overcome cancer has been a long battle in the medical field. It is always the researcher's dream to find a medicine which can cure disease without hurting the human body. Natural healing of cancer in humans has been reported in more than 176 cases (Coley, 1976). There is great potential today for using the body's own immune system to fight cancer. Immunostimulating polysaccharides can help our own immune system to fight cancer. In addition, the polysaccharides not only can suppress the metastasis of cancer, but also can decrease the side effects of radiation and chemotherapy.

In this century, our average lifespan has been extened from 50 years to 78 years. Scientists believe that our average lifespan can reach to 110-140 years. The fact is that our immunities is decrease with age. Immunostimulating polysaccharides will play an important role in our future life. With news on AIDS appearing every week, immunostimulating polysaccharides might play an important role in our daily diets.

IV
Interferon-inducing Chinese Herbs

A. Introduction

Interferon has been touted as a potential cancer-treating drug for nearly 30 years. It was discovered in 1957 by Alick Isaacs and Jean Lindenmann, virologists at London's National Institute for Medical Research (Isaacs and Lindenmann, 1957). It first gained major publicity in 1978 when the American Cancer Society awarded scientists two million dollars for interferon research. Interferons are a family of small protein molecules secreted naturally by human cells to fight viral and other infections. There are three types: Leukocytes, or alpha (α), produced by white blood cells; fibroblast, or beta (β), produced by connective tissue cells; and immune interferon, or gamma (γ), produced by T-cells, a specific variety of white blood cells that are part of the immune system.

Nowadays, Acquired Immune Deficiency Syndrome, or AIDS, is the disease of greatest concern to our society. AIDS is caused by a virus. It has been reported that a Chinese herbal formula might prove helpful in the management of AIDS due to the formula's immunostimulating activity (Smith, 1985). Combined treatment with an interferon-inducing herb and interferon has resulted in a two-fold increase in efficiency on treatment of cervical erosion than treatment with interferon alone (Qian, Li, et al, 1987). In this chapter, the author will briefly review interferon, then survey interferon-inducing Chinese herbs. Their values in clinical application and as a preventive medicine will also be discussed.

B. Types of Interferon and Their Properties

Interferons can be divided into three types: alpha, beta and gamma. Table 6 shows the types of interferon and their properties. A different interferon is produced by a different inducer.

Table 6. Human Interferon

Type	Alpha	Beta	Gamma
Major producing cells	Leucopytes Lymphocytes	Fibroblast	T-lymphocytes
Major inducer	Sendai virus	Double stranded RNA (poly I:C)	Phytohemag-glutin staphylo. enterotoxin
Molecular weight	15,000 & 22,000	24,000	17,000-60,000
Molecular species	>14	1(?)	1(?)
Number of Amino Acids	166	166	146
At pH 2	stable	stable	stable
At 56 degrees C	stable	unstable	unstable
Isoelectric point	5-7	6.5	8.6-8.7

C. Comparison of Interferon, Antibody, and Cellular Immunity

Antibody is defined as humoral immunity which appears in the blood of globulins known as immunoglobulins after vaccination or infection. In contrast, cellular immunity or cell-mediated immunity is concerned with the activity of cells known as T-lymphocytes, which are capable of destroying specific foreign entities such as bacteria and virus. T-lymphocytes play an important role in the prevention of many viral infections. The graft versus host reaction, such as when a patient rejects a transplant - or when a transplant rejects the host - is a cellular immune response. Cellular immunity cannot be transferred by serum, but must be achieved by tranferring actual lymphocytes to the recipients. The differences in biological activities among interferon, antibody, and cellular immunity is summarized in Table 7.

Table 7. Comparison of the Biological Activities of Interferon, Antibody and Cellular Immunity

Interferon	Antibody	Cellular Immunity
Acts on cells and intracellular processes	Directly acts on virus. Does not affect cell.	Acts on infected cells, destroying the infected or cancer cells.
Non-specific	Specific	Specific plus some non-specific functions.
Species-specific	Non-species-specific	Species-specific
Develops in ca. 1-2 days, short-lived	Develops in ca. 2 weeks, permanent	Develops in ca. 2 weeks, permanent

D. Which Tissues Produce the Most Interferon?

Endotoxin was injected into rabbits to examine the respective production of interferon in each tissue. Macrophages, great omentum, liver, spleen, and lymphocytes were found to be the major interferon-producing cells, using endotoxin as the inducer (Kojima, 1984).

E. The Chemical Nature of Interferon-inducer

What type of interferon is going to be produced depends on the chemical nature of the inducer. As I mentioned in Table 6, Sendai virus induces α-interferon production from leukocytes or macrophages and β-interferon is induced by Poly I:C. Phytohemagglutinin stimulates T-lymphocytes to produce γ-interferon. After the discovery of interferon, Isaacs and his associates thought the nucleic acid in the virus was the substance to induce interferon (Isaacs, Cox et al, 1963; Rotem, Cox, Isaacs, 1963). However, this idea was not proved until Hilleman and his associates found that synthetic double-stranded RNA can induce interferon production in addition to viral RNA (Field, Tytell et al, 1967). Many interferon inducers other than nucleic acid have been reported since the late 1960s. The interferon inducers are summarized in Table 8.

The major problems in interferon inducers so far are toxicity and immunological tolerance. Immunological tolerance is defined as when the body is no longer responding to the interferon inducer to produce interferon. The high toxicity and easily developed immunological tolerance in synthetic compounds and microbe-derived interferon inducers cause these difficulties in clinical use.

F. Interferon-inducing Chinese Herbs

Chinese herbal medicines have been used in Asian countries for more than 3,000 years. Most Chinese herbal medicine consists of immunostimulating herbs known to be non-toxic and without side-effects. Herbal formulas are usually taken orally. If a strong interferon-inducing substance among the traditional Chinese herbs can be found, it might be used as a preventive medicine in our daily life or may be deveolped into a non-toxic drug for clinical use without side-effects. Table 9 shows the herbs now known to possess interferon-inducing activity.

Table 8. Interferon Inducers

Microbes and their components	Synthetic Compounds

Virus
   DNA viruses
   DNA viruses
	1. Anionic high molecular
	   weight compounds
	a) Double-stranded RNA such
	   as poly I; poly C

Bacteria	b) Plastic compound containing carboxyl group.
Bordetella pertussis	c) Acidic polysaccharides
Brucella abortus	2. Cationic small molecular
Escherichia coli	weight
Francisella tularensis	compounds
Haemophilus influenzae	a) Tilorone
Klebsicella pneumoniae	b) BL-20803
Listeria monocytogenes	c) CP-20961
Salmonella typhimurium	
Serratia coli	
E. coli Endotoxin	
Brucella abortus Endotoxin	
Salmonella entertidis Endotoxin	

Fungi Components
   Double-Stranded RNA
   Acidic Polysaccharides
   Cationic Low Molecular Substance	

Protozoa
   Toxoplasma gondii
   Plasmodium berghei	

Mitrogen Phytohemagglutinin	

Table 9. Interferon-inducing Chinese Herbs

Appinia offecinarum	Alpinia oxyphylla
Amomum villosum	Angelica dahurica
Angelica sinensis	Aquilaria sinensis
Arctium lappa	Areca catechu
Artemisia capillaris	Artemisia orgyi
Asarum heterotropoides	Asparagus lucidus
Aster tataricus	Astragalus membranaceus
Atractylodes ovata	Benincasa cerifera
Bupleurum chinensis	Carthamus tinctorius
Cimicifuga heracocifolia	Cnidium monnieri
Coriolus versicolor Quel	Corydalis balbosa
Crodus sativa	Cryptotympana atrata
Curcuma zedoaria	Cyperus rotundus L.
Dendrobium officinale	Eucommia ulmoides
Euphorbia kansui	Evodiae fructus
Foeniculum vulgare	Gastrodia elata
Gentiana macrophylla	Hordeum vulgare L. var. hexastion
Houttuynia cordata	Ligusticum chuaxiong
Lindera strychnofolia	Lithospermum crythrorhizon
Lonicera japonica	Magnolia fargesii
Morus alba L.	Notopterygium incisium
Perilla frutescens	Phyllostachys nigra
Pinellia ternata	Plantago asiatica
Polygala tenufolia	Rheum palmatum
Scrophularia ningpoensis	Sinomenium acutum
Sophora augustifolia	Sophora subprostrata
Trachycarpus fortunei	Trichosanthes kirilowii (root)
Trigonella foenum-graecum	Vitex rotundifolia
Xanthium strumarium	Zingiberis officinale (dry)
Zingiberis officinale (raw)	

Among the interferon-inducing Chinese herbs, Angelica dahurica, Angelica sinensis, Benincasa cerifera, Carthamus tinctorius, Curcuma zedoaria, and Morus alba L. showed higher interferon- inducing activity (Kojima, 1984).

Interferon-inducing Chinese herbs are also classified according to the type of interferon that they induce (Table 10). Some herbs show the ability to induce more than one type of interferon, and these include Astralagus membranaceus, Dioscorea batatas, Ganoderma lucidum, and Panax ginseng Meyer (Meng, 1983).

Table 10. Classification of Interferon-inducing Chinnese Herbs According to Type of Interferon

α-interferon	Codonopsis radix	Lentinus edode
	Ganoderma lucidum	Indigo pulverata levis
	Astractylodes ovata	Dioscorea batatas
	Poria cocos	Polyporus umbellatus
β-interferon	Astragalus membranaceus	Panax ginseng Meyer
	Agkistrodon halys	
γ-interferon	Scutellaria baicalensis	Coptis chinensis
	Rehmannia glutinosa	Lonicera japonica
	Taraxicum mongolicum	Viola Yedoensis
	Schizandra chinensis	Paeonia lactiflora
	Cuscuta chinensis	Camptotheca acuminata
	Cucumis melo	Morinda officinalis
	Polygonum multiflorum	Polygonatum officinalis
	Dioscorea batatas	Lycium chinensis
	Panax ginseng Meyer	Astragalus membranaceus
	Ganoderma Lucidum	Glycyrrhiza uralensis

(Meng, 1983)

G. Possible Polysaccharide Structure for Interferon-inducing Activity

It has been shown that interferon-inducing polysaccharide fraction contains a large amount of arabinose. The molar ratio of component sugar arabinose, glucose, galactose, and rhamnose is 12.1:1.0:4.0:1.0. (Yamada, Kiyohara et al, 1984). The interferon-inducing polysaccharide fraction from the seed of Benincasa cerifera showed that the major component sugars are glucose, galactose and galacturonic acid. (Tamamura, Shibukawa, Kojima, 1984). They suggest that the benincasa interferon-inducing polysaccharide consists of $\alpha(1\rightarrow4)$, $\alpha(1\rightarrow6)$ linkage in the structure after treating with dextranase, α-amylase, β-1,3 glucanase, cellulase and concanavalin A.

H. Concluding Remarks

Interferon-inducing activity in many Chinese herbs have also been identified. Since synthetic and microbe-derived interferons have high toxicity and easily develop immunological tolerance, the development of interferon inducers from Chinese herbs might be a better source for this field. Immunities decrease with age, and our average lifespan is increasing. In order to maintain a healthy, happy life, it might be a good idea to employ immunostimulating Chinese herbs in our daily life to boost our immune system, thus enhancing our own natural defense mechanism. With news on AIDS appearing every week, the search for drugs capable of fighting AIDS in prevention or treatment is urgently needed. The interferon-inducing Chinese herbs might provide some answers for this need.

V
Aging, Immunity and Chinese Herbs

A. Introduction

Everything living, without exception, experiences the aging process. Aging is the process toward inevitable death. During this process, many things can happen to shorten life, and these things occur more frequently as aging progresses. Cancer, diabetes, atherosclerosis, hypertension, nephrosis, and Alzheimer's disease are typical diseases associated with the aging process.

Many factors, such as nutrition, health, and material well-being, environment and inheritance can influence the aging process. If we can control diseases of aging while maintaining ideal conditions for health, then survival curves will resemble curve A in Figure 2. To

Figure 2.

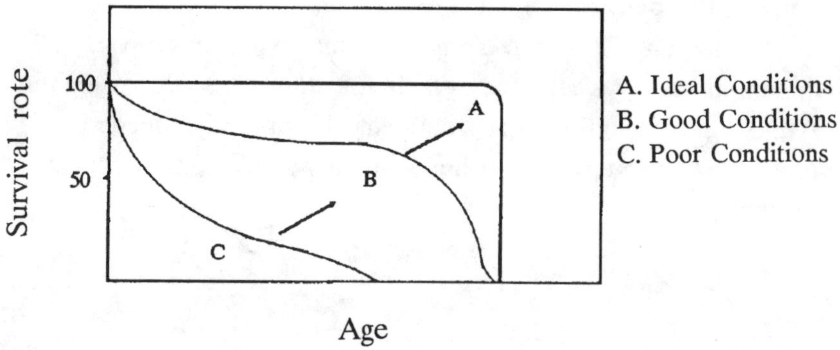

A. Ideal Conditions
B. Good Conditions
C. Poor Conditions

reach the ideal condition of curve A, the present lifespan situation, curve C, will move toward curve B, and in a world of perfect health, finally approach curve A. While it is considered possible to move curve C to curve A, it is generally thought to be impossible to extend curve A further toward the right side of the graph.

The maximum lifespans of different mammals are shown in Table 11.

Table 11. The Mammalian Lifespans

Species	Maximum Lifespan	Species	Maximum Lifespan
Mouse	8	Monkey	35
Horse	46	Cow	30
Orangutan	54	Dog	27
Gorilla	40	Elephant	70
Chimpanzee	45	Man	114

(From Allman and Dittner eds., The Biology Data Book. 1972).

Eternal youth has been an active human quest since ancient times. The First Emperor of the Chin dynesty Ch'in Shih Huang, in about 214 B.C., even sent 500 men and 500 women overseas to look for such an elixir.

How long can we live? Scientists believe that our maximum lifespan is about 110 to 140 years. The oldest documented person died at the age of 116. In this century alone, the average human lifespan has been extended from 50 to 78 years in Japan. The average human lifespan of U.S.A. and European countries are very close to this figure. Improved standards of living, including better nutrition and sanitary conditions, have enabled more of us to live longer. But how can we pass our added years in reasonably good health, in happiness, and in possession of both mental and physical vitality? This chapter will discuss immunological theories of aging and explore what happens to our bodies over time. It will also address the use of Chinese herbal formulas to slow down the effects of aging, and to treat aging-associated disorders.

B. Immunological Theories of Aging

Many researchers have proposed that aging may be related to the well-known fact of the aging body's declining immune response (Burnet, 1959; Comfort, 1964; Walford, 1969, 1974; Makinodan and Adler, 1975). Conditions of cancer, atherosclerosis, hypertension, diabetes, nephrosis, rheumatoid arthritis, and Alzheimer's disease are generally observed in old age.

Some of the body's immunoglobulin (Ig) components are IgA, IgM, and IgG. Increase in IgG levels promotes the possibility of chronic inflammation. IgA level also increases with age, but levels of IgM, which is the first antibody produced immediately after an antigen stimulates a primary immune response, decrease with age. This decrease results in a weakened first line of defense against bacterial infection for elderly people.

The level of the blood's immunosubstance, gamma-globulin, increases with age (Walford, 1969). The increase of gamma- globulin in elderly people results in an increase in autoantibodies (Hooper, 1972). An individual's immune system is normally able to distinguish between its own bodily material and any foreign substance, and normally the body does not initiate an immune response against itself. However, this natural distinction may be disturbed by an overproduction of gamma-globulin, resulting in development of autoantibodies which react against the self, as is seen in autoimmune diseases. Some autoimmune diseases are Addison's diseases, rheumatoid arthritis, thyroiditis, anemia, and systemic lupus erythematosus. There is a correspondence between the occurrence of autoimmune disease and cancer in elderly people. Enhancement of immune system functioning is a pivotal subject in our approach to controlling the debilities of age.

C. Anti-oxidant and Aging

Living cells produce free radicals as part of the metabolism of oxygen for their respiration. Most free radicals are quenched by self-protective systems in our body. However, overproduction of free radicals causes damage in various biomembranes by attacking the unsaturated fatty acids of the biomembranes. Biomembrane damage caused by free radical reactions is believed to be the cause of various aging-associated diseases. Anti-oxidants are the substances which can reduce the free radical reaction or quench free radicals.

Free radicals also cause lipids and proteins to link together. The result is inactive polymers, which are of little use to the cells in which they accumulate (Gedick and Fischer, 1959), but can interfere with the cell's activity. Lipid protein complexes of this type have long been observed in cells throughout the body, and are called "age pigment" or lipofuscin (Stubel, 1911). Hamper (1934) has demonstrated that such complexes of lipid and protein are present in many cell types, and other research has shown that the lipofuscin content of most tissues increases with age (Deane and fawcett, 1952; Sulkin, 1955; Blackett and Hall, 1981).

Ginseng root, ginger rhizome, cimicifuga rhizome, alisma rhizome, liriopes tuber (Han, Han, et al, 1985) and Ganoderma capense (Chen, Wang et al, 1986) have all been found to have anti-oxidant activity.

D. Immunostimulating Chinese Herbs and Chinese Herbal Formulas

We know that the immune system plays an important part in aging. It is definitely possible to enhance the functioning of the immune system through the regular use of single Chinese herbs or Chinese herbal formulas.

1. Immunostimulating Polysaccharides Isolated from Chinese Herbs

Decreased immunity can result in many diseases, such as cancer, diabetes, arthritis, nephrosis and lingering infections. This is why those diseases are associated with aging. It has been known that many Chinese herbs can stimulate immune responses. The major component of immunostimulants have been identified in nature as the polysaccharides (Tsung and Hsu, 1986). The immunostimulating polysaccharides isolated from Chinese herbs have shown β-$(1\rightarrow3)$ and β-$(1\rightarrow6)$ linkages in the polysaccharide structure (Tsung, 1987). Table 12 gives Chinese herbs in which immunostimulating polysaccharides have been isolated (Tsung, 1987).

The functions of the polysaccharides include intensified phagocytosis of reticulocndothelial systems, activation of macrophages, activation of T-lymphocytes, enhancement of cell-mediated immune response, and activation of the alternative pathway of the complement system.

The polysaccharide lentinan isolated from lentinus edodes has been extensively studied for its immunostimulating mechanisms (Tsung, 1987).

Table 12: Chinese Herbs Containing Immunostimulating Polysaccharides

Acanthopanax senticosus	Angelica sinensis
Astragalus mongholicus	Artemisiae argyi
Codonopsis tangshen	Coix lachryma-jobi
Cordyceps ophioglossoides	Coriolus versicolor
Ganoderma lucidum	Lithospermum euchromum
Lentinus edodes	Oldenlandia diffusa
Omphalia lapidescens	Panax ginseng
Panax Pseudoginseng var.	Polyporus mylittae
Notoginseng Burk	Polyporus umbellatus
Poria cocos	

2.Ginseng

Ginseng has been considered for thousands of years in the Orient to be an "anti-aging" herb. Of the 113 prescriptions in the ancient medical text, " Treatise on Febrile Diseases" (Shang Han Lun), 21 contain ginseng. Throughout the nearly two thousand years since the publication of this text, ginseng root has reigned supreme in the field of Chinese medicine.

Ginseng is the most extensively studied Chinese herb. In recent times, the mystery of ginseng's tonic, adaptogenic and anti-aging properties has been gradually clarified by scientific analysis of its components.

Immunostimulating polysaccharides have been isolated from both Asiatic and Siberian ginseng (Tsung and Hsu, 1986). Such immunostimulating polysaccharides enhance the immune system's vitality and effectiveness, even as we age.

We know that free radicals plays a part in aging. Antioxidant components have also been identified in ginseng root (Han et al, 1985). The antioxidant activity in ginseng can eliminate free radicals, helping prevent tissue damage.

Ginseng saponins also affect cholesterol levels and the metabolism of fats. The American Heart Association has concluded that high levels of cholesterol and saturated fats in our blood and body are strongly related to cardiovascular disease, America's leading cause of death. Saponins, the active components of ginseng, have the effect of lowering fat and cholesterol levels in the blood (Yamamoto, Uemura,et al, 1985). In addition, certain human cancers are strongly associated with dietary fats, particularly cancers of the colon and breast. Dietary fats can induce a free radical reaction inside the body. Ginseng, containing saponins and antioxidant components, as mentioned before, can reduce free radical activity and consequently slow the effects of aging which free radicals produce.

Put another way, ginseng's components help bring about bodily homeostasis. (Homeostasis: a state of physiological equilibrium produced by a balance of functions and of chemical composition within an organism). Ginseng saponins can stimulate RNA and protein synthesis (Oura and Yokozawa, 1966); and ginseng's protein synthesis-stimulating factor has been isolated (Oura, Hirai et al, 1975). Ginseng components other than saponins have also been shown to have a regulatory effect on sugar and fat metabolisms. Ginseng components act as metabolic modulators or "adaptogens" depending on general body health and nutrition.

Ginseng stimulates both the nervous and hormonal systems. Healthy physiological functioning depends on the nervous and hormonal systems for the transfer of information from organ to organ. We know that hormonal secretory functions decrease with age. Ginseng has been shown to stimulate the pituitary gland and adrenal cortex to secrete adrenocorticotropic hormone and corticosterone (Hiai, 1981). Studies have found that ginseng can enhance energy, (Reith, Schotman et al, 1975) strength and endurance, and perceptual powers of the sense organs (Halstead and IIood, 1984).

Enhancement of learning and memory by ginseng extract or saponins has also been demonstrated (Saito, 1976; Petkov, 1978). It is possible that ginseng components stimulate the nervous and endocrine systems to secrete materials for adaptation to environment change. This has led to the exciting concept of "adaptogen." Adoptogen is defined as a substance which increases the ability of the body to adapt, and which only works when it is needed. In other words, it only acts to return the body to normal if it had gone off course.

Ginseng is also known to have an anti-stress effect. When subjected to stress on a frequent or long-term basis, an individual may exhibit symptoms such as ulcers, anxiety, chronic fatigue, neurosis, and heart disease. Modern living is notorious for subjecting people to far more stress than the human body was designed to endure. When its defenses are overworked, the body is drained of vitality, and consequently these symptoms of stress can themselves contribute greatly to shortening the lifespan. Adverse effects of stress involve several organ systems and a series of complex physiological interactions among neurotransmitters neuromodulators, and hormones.

Chinese and Japanese researchers (Saito and Bao, 1986) have reported that ginseng appeares to protect against memory failure and decreases in body temperature induced by stress. Ginseng also protectes against adrenal gland enlargement resulting from stress.

In experiments, mice who were stressed showed disturbances in their sexual activity and reproduction. However, applications of ginseng to the mice had the tendency to normalize their sexual cycles (Saito and Bao, 1986).

Ginseng also exhibits radiation protection effects (Yonezawa, 1985; Yonezawa, Hosokawa et al, 1987). Radiation protection activity of ginseng can combine with radiation therapy for cancer treatment and it will be very beneficial to cancer patients. It will also be beneficial to nuclear power plant employees to take ginseng routinely for their protection. Primary target of the damage is known to be the blood-forming tissues in bone marrow (Yonezawa, Hosokawa et al, 1987). This is the reason that the immune system is seriously damage after radiation. The radiation protection effect of ginseng is due to enhancement of the recovery of blood-forming stem cells in the bone marrow (Yonezawa, Hosokawa et al, 1987). Researchers in the Soviet Union have reported similar results (Brekhman and Mayansky, 1965).

Ginseng has been used to treat diabetes in Asia for over 2,000 years. Petkov (1961) has reported that oral administration of an alcohol extract of ginseng causes a decrease in blood sugar levels. Okuda and Yoshida (1980) have extracted an "insulin-like" peptide from ginseng. Insulin is the substance which controls the sugar metabolism. In diabetic patients, their insulin production or secretion is low. Therefore, they are not able to correct the aberration of sugar metabolism. This is why insulin plays a major role in treating diabetic patients. The therapeutic use of ginseng in Asia can be due to the "insulin-like" peptide in ginseng. Kimura (1980) has found that the blood sugar-lowering component of ginseng is not a saponin, but was observed to enhance insulin release. Saponins are considered the functional components of ginseng. That the blood sugar-lowering component of ginseng is a substance other than a saponin means the existence of functional components other than saponins in ginseng. This substance can stimulate insulin secretion and stabilize insulin by suppression of insulin breakdown. Therefore, this substance can help diabetic patients by enhancing the body's function rather than acting as insulin.

Ginseng's experimental effects against cancer cells can be better understood due to the plant's immunostimulating polysaccharides, which promote the body's immune response (Tsung and Hsu, 1986; Tsung,1987). Ginsenosides, or active components of ginseng, have been shown to increase the concentration of cyclic adenosine monophosphate (cAMP), in the cancer culture medium and cAMP has been demonstrated to suppress cancer cell growth   (Abe, Odashima et al, 1980; Odashima, Nishikawa et al, 1980).

Most of the ancient herbal formulas used to treat gastrointestinal ulcers contain ginseng. Ginseng saponins have been shown to be effective in healing ulceration (Sato, 1981). Ginseng extract has been demonstrated to modulate or regulate gastrointestinal tract secretions (Sato, Kojima et al, 1980). (The word adaptogen was coined to describe such a substance that tended to "fill in the gaps" of the body's chemical balance. Several herbs' active ingredients function in this way.)

Ginseng has long been considered to stimulate sexual desire. In the East, ginseng is also widely used to treat impotence, particularly in the aged. Many elderly Chinese men readily admit that their virility is enhanced partly through the use of ginseng and in the laboratory ginseng has been shown to stimulate sperm production and motility (Ishigami, 1973). Yamamoto, Kumagai et al (1977) have shown that when ginseng saponins are added to reproductive organs during in vitro experiments, DNA and protein synthesis increase. Since sperm is made of DNA and protein, the stimulation of DNA and protein synthesis in the reproductive organs should effect the sperm production. Some sex hormones are protein in nature. Therefore, this result may indicate some stimulatory effects of ginseng on reproductive organs.

3. Angelica Sinensis (Tang-kuei, Dang-Gui)

The root of Angelica sinensis, tang-kuei, has a sweet taste, a strong odor, and is considered to benefit the entire female hormonal system. It has been used by tens of millions of Oriental women to tonify their sex organs and maintain normal reproductive functions. Immunomodulating polysaccharides have also been isolated from tang-kuei (Tsung and Hsu, 1986; Yamada, Cyong et al, 1987). Interferon-iuducing activity also has been demonstrated in tang-kuei extract (Yamada, Cyong et al,1987). The most well-known function of interferons is their antiviral activity. It is therefore that Angelica sinenis not only can tonify sex organs and maintain normal reproductive functions but also can regulate the immune system and produce interferons to fight diseases.

4. Ganoderma lucidum (Ling-Zhi)

Ganoderma lucidum is a type of mushroom belonging to the Polyporaceae family. According to "Shen Nung's Herbal," (Shen Nung Pen Tsao Ching) written about 2,000 years ago during the Han Dynasty, ganoderma has six different pharmacological effects associated with its six different colors. Red ganoderma stimulates the heart, internal organs and brain. Black ganoderma re-adjusts kidney functions and electrolyte imbalance. Blue ganoderma is primarily effective for the eyes and liver and also has a tranquilizing effect. White ganoderma suppresses coughing and stimulates lung and spleen functions. Yellow ganoderma is prescribed to treat stomach and chest diseases as well as disorders caused by exhaustion and overindulgence in food and drink. Purple ganoderma is effective for ear diseases and is also thought to stimulate good muscle, bone and joint functions.

It has been recently reported that varieties of ganoderma can regulate blood pressure (Hsu,1986) and control allergies (Kubo laboratory, 1984), and hypolipemic activity (Peng, 1983). It has become clear through research that the ganoderma mushroom is not a single herbal mecicine, but one possessing different pharmacological effects depending upon subspecies and growth environment.

Pharmacological studies confirm that ganoderma's apparent anti- aging effects can be traced to the immunostimulating polysaccharides with their stimulatory effects on the immune system (Tsung and Hsu, 1986; Tsung, 1987).

Hot water extracts of ganoderma have also yielded evidence of allergy-reducing properties (Kubo Laboratory, 1984), and tea made with ganoderma has been effective as a treatment for nephritis, dermatitis, anaphylactic shock and bronchial asthma (Kubo Laboratory, 1984).

5. Astragalus (Huang-Qi)

Astragalus was first recorded in "Shen Nung's Herbal" about 2,000 years ago as a superior herb. A superior herb is a tonic herb that may be taken for a long duration without a side-effect. Astragalus is one of the most frequently used Chinese herbal tonics. It is the dried root of Astragalus membrenaceus or Astragalus mongholicus of the leguminosae family.

Immunostimulating polysaccharides and many immunostimulating activities have been identified in Astragalus (Geng,1986). Interferon-inducing activity also has been reported in Astragalus (Hou, 1981; Meng,1983; Kojima, 1984; Geng, 1986; Tsung, 1988). Interferons are the small proteins which fight viral and other infections.

6. Other Tonic Herbs

Much scientific evidence indicates that most tonic Chinese herbs turn out to possess immounostimulating activity. For example,immunostimulating polysaccharides have been isolated from codonopsis and poria and interferon-inducing activity has been demonstrated in atractylodes, codonopsis, dendrobium, glycyrrhiza (licorice),lycium, polygonum, rehmannia, and schizandra (References: see Chapters of immunostimulating polysaccharedes and interferon-inducing Chinese herbs).

7. Chinese Herbal Formulas with Herbs That Stimulate the Immune System to Help Slow Down Aging.

The following formulas are considered to be the most popular tonic traditional Chinese herbal formulas. All are rich in antiviral, antioxidant, and immunostimulating herbs in their ingredients.

(a). Ginseng Nutritive Combination (Renshen Yangrong tang)

Ingredients: Ginseng, tang-kuei, peony, rehmannia, hoelen, atractylodes, cinnamon, astragalus, citrus, polygala, schizandra, licorice. This formula was recorded in the medical dictionary of the Sung Dynasty (Tai Ping Huei Min Ho Chi Chu Fang, revised in 1149-1152 A.D.).

(b). Ginseng and Tang-kuei Ten Combination (Shiquan Dabu Tang)

Ingredients: ginseng, astragalus, atractylodes, peony, hoelen, rehmannia, tang-kuei, cnidium, cinnamon, licorice.

First recorded in a medical dictionary of the Sun Dynasty (revised in 1149-1152 A.D.) by Chen Shih-wen and Pei Chung-Yuan, it is effective against verious debilitating disorders. Testing of the formula has also yielded evidence of radiation-protective effect (Yonezawa, Hosokawa, 1987).

(c). Ginseng and Astragalus Combination (Buzhong Yiqi Tang)

Ingredients: astragalus, ginseng, licorice, atractylodes, citrus, tang-kuei, cimicifuga, bupleurum, ginger, jujube.

Ginseng and Astragalus Combination is mentioned in the "Identification of Internal and External Diseases" (Nei Wai shang Pien

Huo Lun) by Li Kao in the Yuan Dynasty (1206-1368 A.D.). This formula acts as a tonic for bodily strength and endurance, and has the nickname "king of combinations."

(d). Rehmannia Eight Formula (Bawei Dehuang Wan)

Ingredients: rehmannia, cinnamon, aconite, hoelen, dioscorea, alisma, moutan, cornus.

This formula was recorded in "Prescriptions from Golden Chamber" (Chin Kuei Yao Lueh, 205 A.D.). It can actually reactivate functioning in degenerated kidneys, adrenals and reproductive organs, and it is effective as a preventive and remedy for senility. This formula is very popular in Japan among the elderly (Sokai, 1979). Research has shown the formula to be effective in treating senile cataracts (Fujihira, 1977), and it can improve spermatogenesis (Usuki, 1986).

(e). Minor Bupleurum Combination (Xiao Chaihu Tang).

Ingredients: bupleurum, scute, pinellia, ginseng, jujube, licorice, ginger.

Minor Bupleurum Combination was noted in the "Treatise on Febrile Diseases" and "Prescriptions from the Golden Chamber" (Chin Kuei Yao Lueh), both written by Chang Chung-Ching during the Han Dynasty (207 B.C. - 220 A.D.).

This formula is commonly used for the period of recovery from illness. It treats average patients recovering from, or wishing to ward off, common diseases such as colds, bronchitis and gastric disorders. It is popular as a daily tea in Japan and Taiwan among elderly people.

Minor Bupleurum Combination is used throughout Asia against the common cold and to generally strengthen one against disease.

(f). Ginseng 5 formula

Ingredients: Ginseng, Licorice, Atractylodes, Ginger, Lithospermum.

Lithospermum is added to the ancient formula jen-sheng-tang to meet the demands of today. Lithospermum is the most potent Anti- AIDS virus Chinese herb (Chang and Yeung, 1988). Jen-sheng-tang is recorded in the" Treatise on Febrile Diseases" and "Prescriptions from the Golden Chamber" as a tonic formula.

Ginseng contains immunostimulating polysaccharides, anti-oxidant components and radiation-protective components. Licorice has activiral, interferon-inducing activities and T-cell activation effect. Ginger possesses anti-oxidant components and stimulating effect on clearing circulating immune complexes. Atractylodes has interferon-inducing and anti-cancer activities. Both licorice and lithospermum possess anti-AIDS virus activity. It is a good immunostimulatory and anti-AIDS virus preventive medicine.

E. Enhancing Effect of Chinese Herbs on Clearing Circulating Immune Complexes (C.I.C)

When the body is exposed to an antigen, a specific antibody is produced to bind the antigen, forming a circulating immune complex, or CIC. The immune response is designed to eliminate or neutralize the antigen. When we age, our immunities decline, so naturally the removal of CICs slows down, causing many diseases associated with aging, such as arthritis (Tsung and Hsu, 1987), neoplastic diseases (Teshima, Wanebo, et al, 1977), hepatitis (Thomas, Villier et al, 1978), asthma (Stendardi, Delespesse et al, 1980), and Behcet's disease (Gupta et al, 1978).

Of the 280 kinds of Chinese herbs studied, 20 have been shown to have an enhancing effect on clearing CICs. Most of the herbs possessing the stimulating effect on clearing CICs contain tannin.

Among the 20 active herbs, rhubarb rhizome has shown the strongest activity (Tanaka, Matsumoto, et al, 1987). Polygonacear, zingiberaceae and Ranunculaceae also possess higher activity. In addition to these herbs, Ganoderma lucidum also show a strong activity in clearing CICs (Tsung, 1987).

F. The Hottest-selling Chinese Herbal Formula in Japan: Minor Bupleurum Combination

Chinese herbal medicines have been incorporated into the Japanese medical care system since 1976. Over the past 12 years, Chinese herbal formulas have grown immensely popular among both physicians and patients, due particularly to the fact that, unlike synthesized drugs, herbal formulas lack harmful side effects. A number of research institutes for Chinese medicine have been built, not only by national and private universities, but by pharmaceutical companies as well. The enthusiasm of the Japanese people for Chinese medicines is so great that in 1984 the Japanese government, in cooperation with the government of the People's Republic of China, helped to sponsor and build the world's largest hospital integrating Chinese and Western therapies and treatment. It is called the Chinese-Japanese Friendship Hospital, and is located in Beijing.

Why the Japanese are so fond of Chinese herbal medicines is primarily due to three things: 1. Herbal formulas are too mild to cause side effects; 2. The formulas both relieve the symptoms, and contain immunostimulating components which actually accelerate recovery; 3. The Japanese enjoy the highest average lifespan in the world. Human immune functions decrease as age increases, particularly after the age of about fifty. Since they produce no side effects, elderly persons use tonic formulas to boost their declining immunity, while younger people use herbal formulas as preventive medicine. In its September 4th, 1987 issue, a prominent Japanese magazine, The Asahi Weekly, wrote that Minor Bupleurum Combination is currently the number-one selling formula in Japan. Its herbs include bupleurum, ginger, ginseng, licorice, pinellia, jujube, and scute. Bupleurum extracts have demonstrated a stimulatory effect on antibody and interferon production in the laboratory. (Antibodies and interferon are produced by the body to combat antigens and disease organisms). Saikosaponins isolated from bupleurum have pronounced anti-viral effect, particularly against influenza virus.

Ginseng has been considered to be an "anti-aging" herb in the Orient for thousands of years. Its immunostimulating polysaccharides assist the immune system's function against invading antigens. Antioxidant components in ginseng can also slow down the cellular aging process caused by free radicals. Ginseng saponins affect cholesterol levels and the metabolism of fats. Ginseng's active constituents act as "adaptogens", which "normalize" body functions from conditions of excess, whether high or low. It has also been found that ginseng contains a blood sugar-lowering component.

Ginger stimulates phagocytic activity against infection and toxic substances. Licorice contains glycyrrhizin, which is anti-viral and anti-atherosclerotic, and its extract has shown a stimulative effect on immune response and the production of immunological memory cells. Pinellia can induce production of interferon: small protein molecules secreted by human cells which fight viral and other infections. Jujube and scute have both exhibited anti- allergic effects.

Minor Bupleurum Combination (MBC) is the most frequently used medicine to prevent the common cold in Japan and is traditionally recommended for periods of recovery from illness. It is primarily used by the Japanese as an immunostimulant. Treatment of Acquired Immune Deficiency Syndrome (AIDS) with MBC and other Chinese herbal formulas has been taking place in Japan and the results have been encouraging. The author feels there is a good chance that Minor Bupleurum Combination will soon be a bestselling Chinese herbal formula in the United States.

Japan's Five Most Popular Herbal Formulas

1. Minor Bupleurum Combination

2. Pueraria Combination

3. Cinnamon & Hoelen Formula

4. Rehmannia Eight Formula

5. Minor Blue Dragon Combination

Survey for the Association for Traditional Sino-Japanese Medicine (Nihon Toyo Igakkai), 1987.

G. Concluding Remarks

U.S. life expectancy has risen to a record high of 74.8 years, according to the 1988 report by the National Center for Health Statistics. We know that immunities decrease with age and that decreased immunities can result in the contraction of diseases.

Using immunostimulating, interferon-inducing, antiviral, and anti-oxidant containing Chinese herbs in our daily diets can not only boost our immunities against diseases, but also keep us younger for a happier, healthier life. Therefore, using these Chinese herbs as preventive medicines will be very beneficial.

VI
Allergy and
Chinese Herbs

A. Introduction

An allergy, in plain English, is an out-of-the-ordinary sensitivity to substances that do not bother most people. Most people can tolerate normal amounts of dust around the house, but dust, pollen, molds, fur, and foods such as tomatoes or seafood are only a few of the everyday items to which people can be allergic. Millions of Americans suffer from a runny nose, watery eyes, sneezing fits, hives, the rash of eczema, and the wheezing and shortness of breath of asthma.

Half the people in the world have allergies, and life with an allergy becomes an obstacle course of triggers to avoid. Millions of days are lost from work and school each year because of allergic symptoms, and billions of dollars are spent annually for medical care of allergic patients.

Antihistamine and steroid drugs alleviate allergies. However, antihistamine drugs leave most people too groggy to think straight. Antihistamines also have a side effect which leaves small children and older people restless and unable to sleep. After awhile, antihistamines lose their effectiveness and you have to take more and more of them to obtain the same level of relief. Even though steroid drugs can ease arthritis pain and suppress symptoms of atopic dermatitis, eczema itching and muscle aches, the serious complications which may result from prolonged therapy with steroids include fluid and electorlyte disturbances; hyperglycemia and glycosuria; susceptibility to infections, including tuberculosis; peptic ulcers, which may bleed or perforate; osteoporosis; a characteristic myopathy; psychosis; and Cushing's syndrome, characterized by "moon face," "buffalo hump," supraclavicular fat pads, "central obesity," striae, ecchymoses, acne, and hirsutism.

Since antihistamines and steroid drugs for allergies have hazardous side effects, Chinese herbal medicines have gained more popularity in recent years. The Japanese are already using Chinese herbal medicines to treat allergies with remarkable success. Many Chinese herbal medicines have been approved for use in Japanese physician's prescriptions and are covered by the Japanese National Health Insurance.

The discovery of the effectiveness of ganoderma in allergies has also contributed to the Chinese herbal medicine boom in Japan, mainland China, Taiwan, and other Asian countries.

The author believes it is important that both the public in general and American physicians in particular become informed that many Chinese herbal medicines are effective in the treatment of allergies.

B. What are Allergies?

1. Allergy

The role of the immune system in the body is to identify, capture, destroy and eliminate the "non-self" in order to protect the "self." In the process of elimination of the foreign element, inflammatory reactions and fever will occur in the body with some accompanying damage. Allergy is an immune response that produces tissue injury upon subsequent exposure, even to an agent that is not intrinsically harmful. Like all immune responses, allergies display specificity and memory. Often the damage simply results from an "inappropriate" response; sometimes, but not always, the damage is caused by an excessive response. Here we shall use the term "allergy" to mean "a damaging immune response to an environmental antigen." Antigens that trigger allergic responses are often called allergens.

2. Classification of Allergic Responses and their Pathological Disorders

Allergic responses can be classified as belonging to four to five types(see table 13).

Table 13. Classification of Allergic Responses And Their Pathological Disorders

Classification	Mechanism	Antibody Or Cells	Pathological Disorders
TYPE I immediate allergies	Release of vasoactive substances from antigen-sensitized mast cell; mediated by reaginic antibodies	IgE	Drug allergies; hay fever, hives, bronchial asthma
TYPE II Antibody-mediated cytotoxicity	Cell damage caused by antibodies directed against cell-surface antigens	IgG IgM	Hemolytic disease of the newborn; Goodpasture's syndrome; auto-immune disorders; immune thrombocytopenic purpura

TYPE III Immune complex disorders	Deposits of antigen-antibody complexes activate complement pathway causing inflammation and other tissue damage	lgG lgM	Serum sickness; extrinsic allergic alveolitis; rheumatoid arthritis; chronic hepatitis
TYPE IV Cell-mediated allergies	T-lymphocytes interact with antigen and liberate lymphokines which recruit macrophages to the site	T lymphocytes	Contact dermatitis; tubercular lesions; chronic hepatitis; autoimmune disorders; Hashimoto thyroiditis
TYPE V Anti-receptor	Antibodies directed against cell-surface antigens or receptors alter the physiology of the cell without destroying the cell	lgG	Grave's Disease (thyrotoxicosis)

TYPE I. Immediate Allergies

These are sudden allergic responses mediated by IgE which leads to the release of chemical mediators from mast cells. They are called "immediate allergies" because the allergic response occurs within an hour.

TYPE II. Antibody-mediated Cytotoxicity

Type II reactions produce cell damage which is mediated by complement-fixing antibodies directed against cell-surface antigens. However, antibodies directed against some cell-surface antigens do not kill the cell but instead alter its physiological activity (see Type V).

TYPE III. Immune Complex Disorders

The tissue damage in type III allergies is caused by activation of th complement system following the formation of antigen- antibody complexes.

TYPE IV. Cell-mediated Allergies

These are reactions mediated by T-lymphocytes. Type IV allergies can be differentiated from other types in that there is no involvement of antibodies. They are sometimes called "delayed-type allergies" because the responses take 24-48 hours to appear.

TYPE V. Anti-receptor Antibodies

Type V can be categorized as a subtype of type II. Anti-bodies directed against some cell-surface antigens (hormone receptors, chemical communication receptors) do not kill the cell but instead alter its physiological activity.

C. Anti-allergic Activity of Chinese Herbs

1. The Developing Process of Type I Allergies

Type I allergic responses include such pathological disorders as drug allergies, hay fever, hives, and allergic asthma. The responses are induced immediately by the circulated immunoglobulin E (IgE) attached to mast cells, which releases chemical mediators. In this chapter, the detailed processes or stages of Type I allergic responses will be discussed, together with the efficacy of Chinese herbal formulas in each stage of the allergic response. Type I allergic responses can be divided into three stages (see Fig.3).

Figure 3. The Developing Process Of Type I Allergic Responses

1ST STAGE	1. Invasion of antigen (protein, polysaccharides, lipids, nucleic acid) 2. Production of antibodies (IgE, reagin, anaphylaxic antibody) 3. Antibody attack on mast cells or basophils

2ND STAGE	4. Invasion of antigen 5. Antigen-antibody (IgE) reaction -2 molecules of IgE will bind to 1 molecule of antigen on the target cell -Altered membrane fluidity of the target cell, cGMP($\uparrow$), cAMP($\downarrow$), Ca^{2+}, energy 6. Release of chemical mediators histamine, SRS-A, PC, ECF-A, PAF, NCF

3RD STAGE	7.Pharmacologic reaction of chemical mediator
	    -Symptom names differ according to their position (bronchial asthma, hives, hay fever)
	    -Increased capillary permeability
	    -Contraction of smooth muscle
	    -Hyperthyroid condition
	8. Symptoms

SRS-A = Slow-reacting substance of anaphylaxis
PG = Prostaglandin
ECFA = Eosinophils chemotactic factor of anaphylaxis
PAF = Platelet-activating factor
NCF = Neutrophil chemotactic factor

Since Type I allergic responses can be divided into eight steps in three stages, anti-allergic drugs which suppress the reaction of each step are necessary.

a. The Anti-allergic Substances from Chinese Herbs for the First-stage Response

(i) Treatment by Specific Desensitization

Allergic response will occur when IgE is involved in the elimination of antigens. In order to eliminate the involvement of IgE in the antigen-antibody reaction, stimulation of the production of IgG or IgM is necessary. IgG or IgM can then act as a feedback factor to bring down the level of IgE.

(ii) Anti-allergic Activity of Chinese Herbs

Active investigation of anti-allergic activity in Chinese medicinal herbs has been carried out in many countries.

The herbs which are capable of suppressing IgE activity are licorice, bupleurum, tang-kuei, alisma, jujube, apricot seed, gentiana, cardamom, and Japanese ginseng.(Kohda et al, 1973; Kumagai and Takada, 1974; Nakajima et al, 1980).

Jujube (Zizyphi fructus) has been used as a medicine not just in China, but in Europe, Africa, India, the Middle East, and Australia. It contains cyclic adenosine monophosphate (cAMP) which has a regulatory effect on allergies. (Cyong and Hanabusa, 1980; Hanabusa et al, 1981). The extract of jujube also contains a biologically active substance which can enhance the production of cAMP in the body (Cyony and Takahashi, 1981). The extract also has a β-adrenergic-like activity (Cyong, 1982) It has been reported that ethyl-α-D-fructofuranoside extracted from jujube has a strong anti-IgE production effect (Shibata, 1977). Advances in biochemical and immunological knowledge and in the use of scientific instruments have now provided us with a better understanding of Chinese medicine's true efficacy on a deeper scientific level.

The commonly used anti-allergic Chinese herbal formulas are Bupleurum and Hoelen Combination and Minor Bupleurum Combination. The ingredients of herbs are shown in Tables 14 and 15.

Table 14

Bupleurum and Hoelen Combination or Chailing Tang

Bupleurum	Hoelen
Pinellia	Scute
Ginseng	Jujube
Ginger	Licorice
Cinnamon	Polyporus
Atractylodes	Alisma

Table 15

Minor Bupleurum Combination or Xiao Chaihu Tang

Bupleurum	Scute
Pinellia	Ginseng
Jujube	Licorice
Ginger	

Traditional prescriptions for the use of herbs in the ingredients bupleurum and scute are anti-inflammative and detoxicative, which dispel chest distention. Pinellia and ginger remove the fluid accumulated in the stomach and cure nausea, vomiting, and loss of appetite. A combination of ginseng, jujube and licorice is a stomachic and relieves the sensation of fullness beneath the heart. Bupleurum nourishes the liver. Alisma, polyporus, hoelen, and atractylodes dispel "stagnant water" in the stomach and intestine, incrcase the flow of urine, and eliminate edema. Cinnamon dispels superficial fever, alleviates flushing, and coordinates the diuretic effects of the other herbs.

This knowledges is based on three thousand years' clinical practice in China and many descriptions need further seientific evidence to prove the description. However, scientific evidence shows that bupleurum, ginger, alisma, licorice, jujube and ginseng are capable of suppressing IgE activity (Kohda et al, 1973; Kumagai and Takada, 1974; Shibata, 1977; Nakajima et al, 1980). IgE or immunoglobulin E is the substance causing the release of histamine and other chemical mediators from mast cells which cause drug allergies, hay fever, hives, and allergic asthma. Scute and cinnamon can inhibit the histamine release from the mast cells (Kohda, et al, 1970; Kohda 1981). Atractylodes and ginger also have antihistamine activity (Kokuda et al, 1978; Itokawa et al 1980). Immunostimulating polysaccharides are isolated from ginseng, hoelen and polyporus.

With better understanding of the Bupleurum and Hoelen Combination and Minor Bupleurum Combination on a deeper scientific level, we do know now why these two formulas are the most commonly used anti-allergic Chinese herbal formulas.

b. The Anti-allergic Substances from Chinese herbs for the Second-stage Response

The second stage of allergic response is the stage in which IgE binds to the receptor site of mast cells, which leads to the release of chemical mediators from mast cells. Disodium cromoglycate (DSCG) is the most successful anti-allergy drug developed from natural products because it can suppress this mediator release. DSCG suffers from the disadvantage that it cannot be taken orally and must be applied through inhalation to treat asthma. The Chinese herbs which can inhibit the chemical mediator release are scute, asarum, achyranthes, cinnamon bark, ma-huang, magnolia flowers, bezoar, moutan, ching-pi, and sinomenium (Kohda et al, 1970).

Baicalin, baicalein and skullcapflavone II are the active compounds isolated from scute (Kohda, 1981). These compounds inhibits the release of chemical mediator from mast cells.

Baicalein also inhibits cAMP-hydrolyzing phosphodiesterase and 15-hydroxy prostaglandin dehydrogenase, which hydrolyzes prostaglandin E_1. cAMP and prostaglandin E_1 inhibit chemical mediator release.

The most commonly used anti-allergic Chinese herbal formulas in this stage are Minor Bupleurum Combination, Minor Blue Dragon Combination and Ma-huang and Apricot Seed Combination (Kubo and Kotani, 1984).

We have examined the efficacy of Minor Bupleurum Combination on anti-allergic activities in the previous section. Now, we also will examine why Minor Blue Dragon Combination and Ma-huang and Apricot Seed Combination are the popular herbal formulas for the second-stage response of Type I allergies. As shown in Table 16, both combinations contain ma-huang and licorice. Ma-huang inhibits chemical mediator such as histamine from mast cells (Kohda et al, 1970) and licorice has been shown to supperss IgE activity (Kohda et al, 1973; Kumagai and Takada, 1974; Nakajima, et al 1980) and anti-complement activity (Kohda and Nagai, 1974; Shibata, 1980).

Table 16

Ma-huang and Apricot Seed Combination or
Ma xing Gan Shi Tang

Ma-huang	Apricot seed
Licorice	Gypsum

Minor Blue Dragon Combination or Xiao Qinglong Tang

Pinellia	Ma-huang
Peony	Licorice
Cinnamon	Asarum
Schizandra	Ginger

Apricot seed in the ingredients of Ma-huang and Apricot Seed Combination can suppress IgE activity (Kohda et al, 1973; Kumagai and Takeda, 1974; Nakajima, et al 1980). Gypsum is traditionally used as a refrigerant and antipyretic.

In the ingredients of Minor Blue Dragon Combination, asarum, cinnamon, and ginger, inhibit histamine and other chemical mediators from mast cells (Kohda et al, 1970), and Pinellia and Schizandra exhibit anti-inflammatory activity (Kohda, 1986). Peony is antitussive.

From the scientific evidence of Chinese herbs used in the three anti-allergic combinations, it is easy to understand why they are the most commonly used formulas.

C. The Anti-allergic Substances from Chinese Herbs for the Third-stage Response

This is the stage in which chemical mediators mediate the pharmacologic reactions causing the increase in capillary permeability, contraction of smooth muscles, and hyperthyroidism. The symptoms are named according to the part of the body affected: bronchial asthma, allergic rhinitis (hay fever), allergic urticaria (hives), and allergic gastroenteritis. Medicines for this stage should have an inhibitory effect on chemical mediator release or an anti-inflammatory activity. Clinically, beta-adrenergic stimulants and xanthine derivatives are used as bronchodilators for bronchial asthma and anti-histamine drugs are used for hay fever and hives.

Chinese herbs which have an anti-histamine effect are zedoaria, ginger, galanga, cardamom, cluster, and alpinia (Itokawa et al, 1980). Beta-eudesmol and nerolidol have been identified as the functional compounds from these Chinese herbs (Itokawa et al, 1980). Atractylodes, sinomenium, and asarum also exhibit anti-histamine activity. The functional compounds identified in asarum are methyleugenol and higenamine (Kokuda et al, 1978).

Chinese herbal formulas commonly used as anti-allergic medicines in stage three are Minor Blue Dragon Combination, Pueraria & Magnolia Combination, and Tang-kuei & Arctium Formula.

2. Chinese Herbal Formulas for Type II Allergies

Cell damage produced by type II allergies are mediated by the activation of complements due to complement-fixing antibodies directed against cell-surface antigens.

The allergic symptoms of type II include the side effects of transfusing the wrong blood type, autoimmune hemolytic anemia, hemolytic anemia due to drug allergy, and decrease of platelets. Anti-complement activity has been found in both licorice and cinnamon bark (Kohda and Nagai, 1974; Shibata, 1977). Chinese herb formulas for type II allergies feature mainly these two herbs.

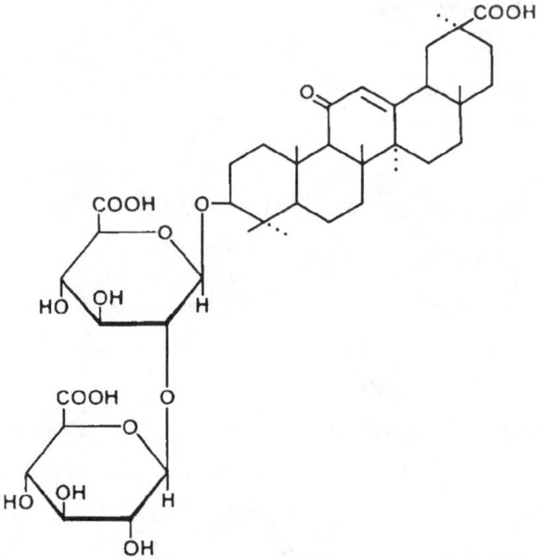

Figure 4. Glycyrrhizin from Licorice

3. Chinese Herbal Formulas for Type III Allergies

Since the tissue damage in type III allergies is caused by activation of the complement system following the formation of antigen-antibodies, the medicines for type III allergies are either anti-complement or anti-inflammatory drugs.

Immune-complex disorders (type III allergies) are bacterial glomerular nephritis, chronic B-type hepatitis, atopic bronchial asthma, erythromatosis, chronic rheumatic arthritis, and thyroiditis.

Chinese herb formulas for immune-complex disorders use herbs prescribed for kidney disorders and are anti-complement and anti-inflammatory. Commonly used formulas are Atractylodes Combination, Bupleurum and Hoelen Combination, Bupleurum and Dragon bone combination, Stephania and Astragalus Combination, and Rehmannia Eight Formula (Kubo and Kotani, 1984).

Saikosaponins have been isolated from bupleurum, and are known to be active components for anti-allergic activity

(Yamamoto, Kumagai, et al, 1975a,b; Shibata 1977, 1980). Yamamoto et al (1975a,b) found that saikosaponins a and d have steroid-type anti-inflammatory action. Saikosaponins b1 and b2 have stronger anti-type III allergic activity than saikosaponins a and d. Fig. 5 shows the chemical structures of saikosaponins from bupleurum.

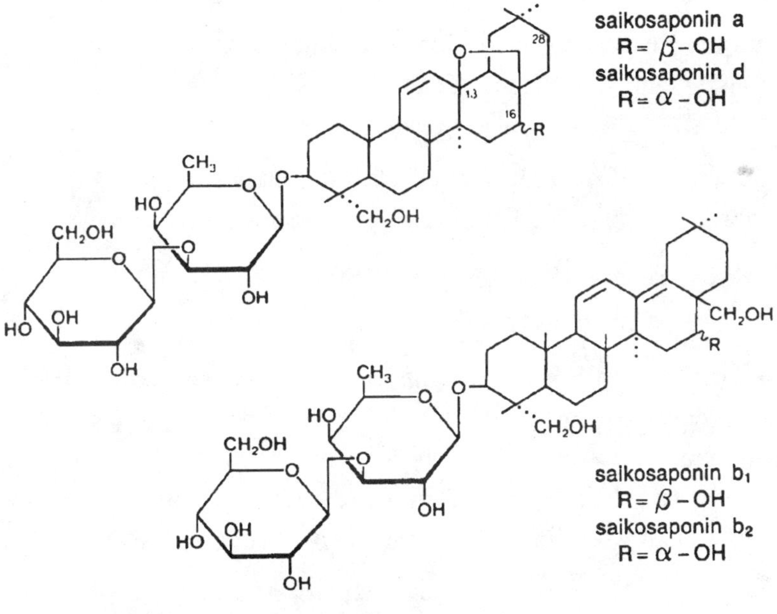

Figure 5. Saikosaponin Structures from Bupleurum

4. Chinese Herbal Formulas for Type IV Allergies

Type IV allergies are different from types I-III in that there is no involvement of antibodies. This type of allergy is mediated by T-lymphocytes. The symptoms are contact dermatitis, tubercular lesions, chronic hepatitis, erythromatosis, rheumatoid arthritis, Hashimoto thyroiditis, and ulcerous intestinitis.

Chinese herbs prescribed for these allergies are ginseng, magnolia bark, hoelen, licorice, pinellia, and jujube,(Kohda et al, 1982; Nishii et al 1982).

Commonly used formulas are Minor Bupleurum Combination, Bupleurum & Hoelen Combination, and Bupleurum & Schizonepeta Combination (Nakajima et al, 1980; Nishii et al, 1982) and Minor Blue Dragon Combination, (Yagi et al, 1980) Cinnamon & Atractylodes Combination, and Tang-kuei & Gardenia Combination (Kotani et al, 1983). Minor Blue Dragon Combination is especially good for bronchial asthma and hay fever. Pueraria Combination and Tang- kuei & Gardenia Combination are effective in treating allergic dermatitis.

Since type V allergies can be classified as a subtype of type II, the herbal formulas for type II allergies are recommended.

5. Enhancement of the Efficacy of Steroid Drugs by Chinese Herbal Formulas

When Magnolia & Bupleurum Combination was combined with a steroid drug to treat contact dermatitis, the efficacy of the steroid was enhanced by the Chinese herbal formula. In fact, the amount of steroid could be decreased by more than half when the steroid was combined with the herbal formula (Kohda et al, 1982).

In the treatment of other allergies, the combination of steroid drugs and Chinese herbal formulas has been shown to enhance the efficacy of the steroid drug in numerous clinical trials (Arichi and Kotani, 1980). The steroid drug dosage can be decreased drastically by combining it with Minor Bupleurum Combination, Bupleurum, Cinnamon & Ginger Combination, or Bupleurum & Cinnamon Combination to treat chronic bronchial asthma (Fujimura and Osada, 1982).

Steroids are very useful drugs for the treatment of allergies and inflammatory diseases. However, steroids also have strong adverse side effects which can be overcome by combining them with Chinese herbal formulas.

D. Anti-Allergic Activity of Ganoderma Lucidum

1. The Discovery of Anti-allergic Ganoderma

Shen Nungs' Herbal stated that white ganoderma had a suppressing effect on coughs. To investigate this claim, the anti-allergic activity of white ganoderma was tested by a Japanese group at Kinki University. They found that the hot-water extract of white ganoderma did have a strong suppressive activity on the histamine release from mast cells (Kubo Lab., 1984). The extract also suppressed the passive cutaneous anaphylaxis (PCA) reaction. In PCA analysis, a sample of the serum to be assayed is injected into the shaved skin of an albino guinea pig. After a period of approximately 24 hours, the antigen is injected intravenously together with a marker, Evan blue dye. Evan blue binds to serum albumin and thus is normally retained within the blood vessels. However, where an antigen meets sensitized mast cells, the release of vasoactive substances increases capillary permeability so that the dye passes into the tissue spaces and the reaction site becomes blue.

Since the ganoderma extract can suppress histamine release from mast cells and suppress PCA reaction, it is expected to do well against type I allergies, including anaphylactic shock, atopic dermatitis and bronchial asthma.

White ganoderma also appears to be effective against such immune-complex disorders as serum sickness, extrinsic allergic alveolitis, rheumatoid arthritis and chronic hepatitis. In the animal model for immune-complex disorders (type III allergies), nephritis is induced by successive injections of rabbit serum protein into rats, causing antigen-antibody complexes to develop in the blood stream and to be deposited in the kidneys. The antigen-antibody complexes deposited in the kidneys are supposed to be phagocytosed and disposed of by the phagocytes in the reticuloendothelial system of the kidney. However, when the flow of antigen-antibody complexes from the blood stream is continuous, the phagocytes are unable to dispose of the complexes and must be helped by the phagocytes, leukocytes and monocytes in the blood stream. The inflammatory reaction thus developed in the kidney is called nephritis. In nephritis, both protein concentration in urine and cholesterol concentration in serum are increased. With treatment by white ganoderma extract, protein and cholesterol concentrations were reduced to normal levels. Morphological observation of the kidney also showed recovery, and hypertension due to nephritis was returned to normal.

White ganoderma extract also did well against such cell-mediated allergies as picryl chloride-induced dermatitis in mice. In addition, the extract showed great enhancement of steroid-drug effect in the treatment of dermatitis. Due, again, to the steroid drugs' considerable side effects, any decrease in steroid dosage is beneficial to patients.

It's also important to isolate the active anti-allergic compounds from ganoderma, because ganoderic acids (see Figure 6) have been found to be one of the components responsible for inhibiting histamine release from mast cells. Since ganoderma has a multiple activity on type I to type V allergies, the active components on different allergic reactions are expected to be different. In order to solve the mystery of the multiple functions of ganoderma, many research groups have been working on this subject in many countries. The puzzle could possibly be solved in the near future.

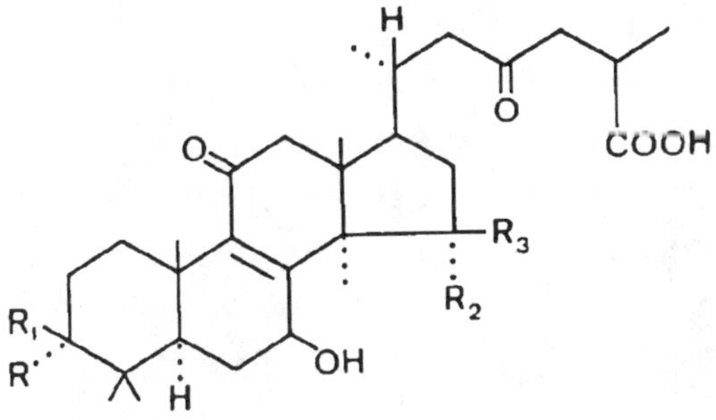

Ganoderic acid A $RR_1 = O$, $R_2 = OH$, $R_3 = H$
Ganoderic acid B $R = OH$, $R_1 = H$, $R_2R_3 = O$

Figure 6. Chemical Structure of Ganoderic Acids

E. Concluding Remarks

Accumulated scientific evidence indicates that the Chinese herbal formulas prescribed for allergies are based on each stage of the allergic reactions. In order for readers to comprehend the scientific basis, the author has introduced as many as possible of the active chemical compounds which have been isolated from Chinese herbs.

The Chinese and Japanese are already using Chinese herbs or Chinese herbal formulas to treat allergies with considerable success. 148 Chinese herbal formulas are approved for use in Japanese physicians' prescriptions and are reimbursed by Japanese National Health Insurance.

The discovery of the effectiveness of ganoderma in all types of allergies gives us hope that powerful new anti-allergic compounds can be isolated from ganoderma.

The combination of Chinese herbal formulas and steroid drugs can in many cases significantly reduce the amount of steroids used, which is very beneficial to patients, since it minimizes side effects.

Most Chinese herbal formulas are designed to relieve painful symptoms and at the same time modulate the immune system to adapt to the condition. All the formulas promote equilibrium of the physical condition and maximum health. This is why Chinese herbal formulas work on the body without side effects. Even though the author has introduced many of the active chemical compounds isolated from Chinese herbs, it does not mean a single chemical compound can substitute for any one of the Chinese formulas.

VII
Arthritis and
Chinese Herbs

A. Introduction

We frequently receive desperate phone calls and letters from arthritis victims who complain about the side effcts of Western medicines and want us to recommend a Chinese medicine to ease their pain. For example, one correspondent wrote: "According to Western medicine the medicine for arthritis is aspirin. Unfortunately, my stomach cannot tolerate aspirin any more. In September 1984, I had major surgery and half of my stomach was cut away. I am looking for the right medicine for my arthritis and would like to have your honest opinion."

Arthritis causes more prolonged pain to more Americans than any other disease. At least seven million Americans are reported to be afficted with constant arthritis pain. Although more than 33 million dollars have been spent on arthritis-related research through the National Institute of Health, an estimated 70 million work-days were lost because of arthritis during the past year and some 500,000 sufferers required hospitalization. The personal tragedies that this involves can only be guessed at from the letters we have received from arthritis victims.

In rheumatoid arthritis, researchers believe that the body's immune system is not working properly. Gout, another form of arthritis, is a disease of metabolic disorder. Arthritis can be called a patient-specific syndrome. Every biologically unique arthritic patient has his or her own body chemistry and immune system which determines his or her particular immune response.

The principle of Chinese medicine is to diagnose symptoms or illnesses in terms of the patient's individuality. Most Chinese herbal formulas are designed not only to relieve symptomatic pain but, more importantly, to enhance the body's immune system by stimulating metabolism and the function of the endocrine system. Therefore, Chinese medicine, as a patient-specific therapy, is well suited to the treatment of arthritis, a patient-specific syndrome.

B. What is Rheumatoid Arthritis?

Rheumatoid arthritis is an inflammatory disease of connective tissue with major symptoms of joint swelling and pain. The initial stage of rheumatoid arthritis is marked by symmetrical swelling and pain in the joints of the fingers, hands, and knees. Gradually, the joints are destroyed and deformed, so that they are less and less able to function. Eventually, the joints become immobile.

It has been suggested that a pathogen-like virus causes the disease. However, there is no strong evidence to support this theory. The theory that it is an autoimmune disorder is supported by two observations: (i) the C-reactive protein in the immunoglobulin fraction is increased in the serum of rheumatoid arthritis patients, and (ii) denatured immunoglobulin (IgG), called "the rheumatoid factor," is increased in the serum of these patients. Therefore, it seems likely that complexes of IgG and anti-IgG antibodies are deposited in the joints, their presence eliciting the inflammatory reactions leading to swelling and pain in the joints. Interleukin-1 is also found in increased concentrations in the joints of rheumatoid arthritis patients. Interleukin-I is a substance released from white cells. Probably Interleukin-I is also strongly linked to rheumatoid arthritis.

C. Western Medicine and Rheumatoid Arthritis

There is no drug that can cure chronic rheumatoid arthritis at the present time. The drugs used for its treatment merely control the symptoms and ease pain by suppressing or masking symptoms. Those most commonly used are steroids, non-steroid, anti-inflammatory drugs, anti-rheumatoid agents and immunosuppressors or immunomodulators.

1. Steroids

Steroids are the most commonly used drugs for arthritis. However, they cannot cure arthritis; they can only ease the pain by suppressing the symptoms. The principal complications resulting from prolonged therapy with steroids are fluid and electrolyte disturbances; hyperglycemia and glycosuria; susceptibility to infections, including tuberculosis; peptic ulcer, which may bleed or perforate; osteoporosis; a characteristic myopathy; psychosis; and Cushing's syndrome, consisting of "moon face," "buffalo hump," supraclavicular fat pads, "central obesity," striae, ecchymoses, acne, and hirsutism.

2. Non-steroid anti-inflammatory drugs

The most common nonsteroid anti-inflammatory drugs are aspirin, phenylbutazone, and idomethacin. These drugs are for short-term usage only. Long-term use of these drugs can result in such complications as gastric ulceration and bleeding, abdominal pain, skin eruptions, CNS disturbances, and disturbance of the acid- base balance and electrolyte structure of blood plasma.

3. Anti-rheumatoid agents

Gold compounds and penicillamine are commonly used anti-rheumatoid agents. These agents are anti-inflammatory, but they have no direct effect upon pain. Although they appear to induce a remission in active rheumatoid arthritis, the drawback of these agents is their potential for damage to the kidneys and blood, which necessitates periodic urine and blood tests.

4. Immunosuppressors and immunomodulators

Anti-cancer drugs which have an immunosuppressive effect have been applied to arthritis treatment (i.e. cyclophosphamide, 6-methylpurine, azathioprine). The usual side effects of immunosuppressors are anorexia, nausea, and vomiting; long-term use may increase the incidence of some cancers, infections and bone marrow suppression. These very dangerous immunosuppressive drugs suppress the body's immune system and the body needs its immune system's protective powers to defend against other illness.

In addition to drug therapy, physical, diet, acupuncture, and surgical therapies have been used.

D. Rheumatoid Arthritis in Chinese Herbal Medicine

In Chinese medicine the term "moisture disease" has no Western medical equivalent, but it has been generally translated as "wind and moisture disease," a phrase which is now commonly used. One of the first references to "wind and moisture disease" appears in "Prescriptions from the Golden Chamber" (Chin kuei yao lueh), where it is used to define an illness accompanied by generalized pain.

Chinese medical theory holds that diseases are brought about by either internal or external causes. External causes arise mainly from geography, weather, and environment, and are known as the "six excesses": wind, dryness, cold, fire, moisture, and heat. Because "wind and moisture fight each other," the patient feels severe bone and joint pain, making it very difficult for him to stretch or bend. As early as "The Yellow Emperor's Treatise on Internal Medicine"; "wind and moisture" was described as one of the "numb diseases" in Chinese medicine. A "numb disease" is characterized by an increase of pain due to cold or damp weather.

E. Chinese Herbal Formulas for Rheumatic Fever and Early-Stage Rheumatoid Arthritis

Rheumatic fever usually starts with an acute inflammation and painful swelling of the joints; before the condition is brought under control, many of its victims are left with permanently damaged hearts. While most cases start with painful swelling in the joints, it is good to remember that the acute inflammatory process does not always limit itself to the joints. The heart, the blood vessels, the kidneys, the nerves, and other organs of the body are often involved, while occasionally the joints themselves are free and clear.

For rheumatic fever and the early stage of rheumatoid arthritis, Ma-huang and Atractylodes Combination and Ma-huang and Coix Combination are commonly used formulas (see Table 17).

Table 17. Ingredients of Ma-huang and AtractylodesCombination (MAC) and Ma-huand and Coix Combination (MCC)

MAC	MCC
Ma-huang	Ma-huang
Apricot seed	Apricot seed
Licorice	Licorice
Cinnamon	Coix
Gypsum	
Atractylodes (white)	

Ma-huang, apricot seed, and licorice are the common components in the two formulas.

Ma-huang contains the chemical compounds ephedrine, pseudo-ephedrine, N-methylephedrine, and N-methyl-pseudoephedrine as its major active components. Ma-huang is considered to have anti-inflammatory activity.

Apricot seed is considered to be an excellent health food for the throat and is commonly used as cough medicine and in the treatment of bronchial asthma. It is also considered to have a mucoregulator function. Vocalists frequently use a drink made from apricot seed to maintain the quality and strength of their voices. Amygdalin (Saito, 1982), β-glucosidase (Kariyone, 1964; Nagoshi and Nakano, 1976; Akabori and Kagawa, 1983), aminopeptidase (Ninomiya, et al 1982), and the steroid compounds estrone and estradiol-β-17-ol (Awad, 1974) have been identified in the apricot seed. However, the pharmacologically active components are not necessarily limited to these materials.

Licorice contains glycyrrhizin, which is known to have anti-inflammatory activity and stimulatory activity in reticuloendothelial systems (Miyake, 1961; Yamauchi and Tsunematsu, 1981/82).

Cinnamon possesses antibacterial properties (Pruthi, 1980), and atractylodes contain anti-histamine compounds β-eudesmol and hinesol (Itokawa, et al, 1980). An infusion of coix is considered nutritive, refrigerant, and diuretic; alcohol fermented from the seeds is considered antirheumatic. Coixol isolated from coix has a muscle-relaxing effect.

Ma-huang and Atractylodes Combination and Ma-huang and Coix Combination are also effective on other forms of arthritis.

F. Chinese Herbal Formulas and Chronic Rheumatoid Arthritis

Because of the hazardous side effects of Western medications, Chinese herbal medicine has become increasingly popular in Japan, Taiwan, and Mainland China for the treatment of chronic rheumatoid arthritis.

Cinnamon and Atractylodes Combination (Guizhi Jia Ling Shu Fu Tang) is the most widely prescribed Chinese herbal medicine in Japan. In cases of rheumatic fever and early-stage rheumatoid arthritis, the prescribed Chinese herbal formulas contain Mahuang as the anti-inflammatory component. However, aconite is the key component in the herbal formulas for chronic rheumatoid arthritis. Aconite content in the formulas is increased according to the stage of the disease; a smaller amount is prescribed for acute rheumatoid arthritis.

Aconite contains aconitine and related alkaloids. The fresh herb is extremely toxic, but in the dried root much of the aconitine has decomposed to picroaconitine and aconine, which are less toxic (Lu, 1954).

Aconite was prescribed in twenty of the fomulas listed in the " Treatise on Febrile Diseases," and in 29 of the formulas in "Prescriptions from the Golden Chamber." Its popularity is due to the stimulatory effect that it has on metabolism and its ability to control pain.

Aconite is used not only in Cinnamon and Atractylodes Combination, Licorice and Aconite Combination (Gancao Fuzi Tang) and other formulas for rheumatoid arthritis, neuralgia, and hemiplegia, but also in Rehmannia Eight Formula (Bawei Dehuang Wan) and other herbal formulas for diseases of old age, e.g. diabetes, lower hack pain, and skin disease, and in Vitality Combination (Zhenwu Tang) for chronic diarrhea.

Cardiotonic effect is also found in aconite. In addition to aconitine and related alkaloids, a cardiotonic compound higenamine (Kosuga et al, 1978) and a hypertensive compound coryneine (Konno et al, 1979) have been isolated from aconite.

The Chinese herbal formulas commonly used in Japan for chronic rhedmatoid arthritis are as follows (Tashiro, 1985):

> Cinnamon and Anemarrhena Combination
> Cinnamon and Atractylodes Combination
> Cinnamon and Hoelen Commbination
> Coix Combination
> Coix Combination with Processed Aconite
> Licorice and Astragalus Combination with Aconite
> Tang-Kuei and Anemarrhena Combination

G. Efficacy of Steroid Drugs With Chinese Herbal Formulas

The combination of steroid drugs and Chinese herbal medicines has also been demonstrated in numerous clinical trials to enhance the efficacy of steroid drugs used in the treatment of arthritis. Although the disadvantages of the potential side effects are obvious, the advantage of steroids in easing pain quickly and for a relatively long period is not to be denied. Fortunately, when certain Chinese herbal formulas are combined with steroids they have been found to minimize the risk of such side effects (Sokai, 1978; Arichi and Kotani, 1980; Kaneko, 1981; Arichi, 1982).

H. Western Medicine and Gout

In Western medicine gout is classified as a joint disease which is characterized by acute arthritic pain in the peripheral joints. The disease is caused by abnormal metabolism of uric acid. In over 95 percent of the cases, the excessive serum urate concentration results in hyperuricemia. The arthritic pain of gout is due to the deposit of uric acid crystals around the joint. Urate deposits may also appear in other parts of the body as tophi. The deposit of monosodium urate crystals in the kidneys, however, may result in serious kidney damage. Excess excretion of uric acid through the kidneys may produce kidney stones (10%-20% of the cases), while deficient excretion may result in hyperuricemia.

Gout often affects those who eat and drink excessively. Most patients are over 40 years old, and about seventy percent are obese. The ratio of male to female patients is 20:1.

There are two types: acute gouty arthritis and chronic gout. The onset of the disease is frequently sudden. The first attack usually occurs at the metatarsophalangeal joint of the great toe, though it may also occur at finger, wrist, ankle, or knee joints. Two to three hours after the pain begins, the joint becomes swollen and excruciatingly tender and the skin turns dark red. Although the joint function returns to normal after the first attack, such episodes may recur after several months or even two years. As the disease progresses, the attacks become more frequent and more severe. Without prophylactic therapy, chronic gout may develop.

The usual therapy for patients with gout is colchicine, a drug derived from the autumn crocus and discovered in ancient Egypt. Since a side effect of colchicine may be acute diarrhea, the drug should be taken only as directed by a physician.

Other drugs which are frequently prescribed for gout are Benemid and Anturan, both of which increase the excretion of uric acid and thereby promptly lower the plasma uric acid level. The side effects are stimulation of the central nervous system, gastrointestinal irritation, convulsions, and possible death from respiratory failure.

I. Chinese Medicine and Gout

In the "Treatise on Febrile Diseases" and "Prescriptions from the Golden Chamber," there is no mention of any term for gout. Since foods were prepared in a simple manner in ancient China, perhaps the disease did not exist. However, during the Yuan Dyanasty, the term for gout appeared in medical documents.

In Chinese medicine, the word for gout means "painful numbness" or "numb pain." According to the medical classics, other terms for gout include "evil wind," "numb disease," "seasonal disease," or "white tiger pain" (since the pain is sharp like a tiger's bite). The symptoms of the disease are acute pain in various joints throughout the body, weakness of both ch'i and blood, and immobility of the joints. If the pain is very acute, the disease is called "white tiger seasonal disease." The use of the various terms for gout in Chinese medicine closely parallels the definitions in modern Western medicine. The so-called "gout of old age" probably refers to gouty arthritis or rheumatism.

According to the principles of Chinese medicine, gout occurs when the "seven sentiments" are attacked by chills, moisture, and wind. The objectives of therapy are regulation of the circulation of ch'i and blood in the blood vessels and relief of the patient's nervous tension.

The most popular formula prescribed by modern Chinese physicians for treating gout is Tang-Kuei and Anemarrhena Combination. This formula serves as an anodyne.

J. Concluding Remarks

The value of Chinese herbal formulas in the treatment of arthritis can be summarized as follows:

(1) Western medicines used for the treatment of arthritis include steroids, non-steroid anti-inflammatory drugs, anti-rheumatoid agents and immunosuppressors or immunomodulators. These drugs can only control the symptoms and ease the pain of arthritis. However, the incidence of hazardous side effects with these drugs is high. In the course of more than 3,000 years of clinical experience with billions of people, a number of Chinese herbal formulas have been developed for the effective treatment of arthritis. The identification of many of their active chemical components during the past fifty years has made it easier for us to understand how Chinese herbs act upon arthritis.

(2) Many Chinese herbal formulas have been approved for use in physicians' prescription in Japan and are covered by Japanese National Health Insurance.

(3) The combination of Chinese herbal medicines and steroid drugs can reduce the amount of steroid to be used by enhancing the steroid effect, which is very beneficial to patients since the side effects of steroids can then be minimized.

(4) I think that it is important that both the public in general and American physicians in particular become aware of the role that Chinese herbal formulas can play in the treatment of arthritis. It is partly for this reason that I have introduced the active chemical compounds isolated from Chinese herbs wherever this evidence is relevant.

(5) I hope that this book will encourage more American physicians to consider the use of Chinese herbal formulas in treating their arthritis patients.

VIII
AIDS and
Chinese Herbs

A. Introduction

Nowadays, it is almost impossible not to have heard and seen the term AIDS (Aquired Immune Deficiency Syndrome) in our daily lives. AIDS has not only become the urgent medical issue but also has become world-wide social issue.

According to the US Center for Disease Control, 85,590 AIDS cases have been diagnosed and 48,957 AIDS deaths have been recorded in the United States as of February 6, 1989.

Scientists are getting to know the AIDS virus in extraordinary detail. But the more they learn, the more discouraged they are about the prospects for rapidly finding a cure or vaccine. The virus, formally known as the human immunodeficiency virus or HIV, attacks the body in more ways than had been suspected, and in more devious ways.

Since the only FDA-approved drug azidothymidine (AZT), has a severe side-effect and limited availability, many AIDS communities and physicians are using Chinese herbs for AIDS treatment since anti-HIV activity has been found in Chinese herbs (Ito, Nakashima, Baba et al, 1987; Chang and Yeung, 1988; Meruelo, Lavie, and Lavie, 1988). In this chapter, the studies of herbs on AIDS will be discussed.

B. How the AIDS Virus Infects our Bodies?

Scientists thought that the AIDS virus, like many others, was transmitted as a virus particle in blood, semen or vaginal fluid. However, researchers have found that the main source of AIDS virus in semen and vaginal fluid is not free virus particles, but virus-carrying macrophages in those fluids.

Macrophages are phagocytic cells in the immune system that collect and carry substances throughout the body. The AIDS virus is picked up by macrophages and carried in special sacs. Once hidden in these sacs, the virus is undetectable by the antibody. The antibody is an immunoglobulin molecule that interacts with the antigen. In this case, the antigen is the AIDS virus. Therefore, a vaccine may not be effective against the virus carried in macrophages. Macrophages can carry the AIDS virus to other parts of the body, enabling the virus to infect cells. Macrophages also can pass the AIDS virus to T-lymphocytes or T-cells. T-cells are immune cells that normally activate the body's defences against diseases. Unlike the macrophages, T-cells die when they release the virus, leading to the eventual destruction of the immune system. Killing the macrophages may not stop their destructive cycle because the AIDS virus is relsesed when the macrophage dies.

A new study also has found that the AIDS virus can infect and grow in very immature bone marrow cells, which show no characteristics of the mature cells they will eventually become. As they mature, these cells change dramatically and turn into monocytes and macrophages, scavenger cells of the immune system. Infected monocytes and macrophages may fail to fight infections and may spread the virus to other immune system cells.

As the AIDS virus grow inside the bone marrow cells and the cells accumulate huge numbers of viruses inside them, the cells show no exterior signs of infection. This means that the virus can reproduce itself without showing itself to the immune system to be destroyed.

It is not sure how the virus originally enters these immature cells. Ordinarilly, the virus latches onto a protein, CD-4, that is on the surface of immune system cells, and the CD-4 protein pulls the virus in. But researchers could not find CD-4 on the surfaces of immature cells, although it is possible that small numbers of CD-4 proteins were present but eluded detection. The researchers found that as the marrow cells matured, and after they were infected, CD-4 proteins began appearing on their surfaces.

The way the virus grows in the immature marrow cells resembles its growth in monocytes and macrophages. The virus accumulates inside the cells but does not burst out. There are indications that this sort of growth pattern may render the virus more resistant to AZT, the only drug to receive Federal approval for fighting AIDS infections.

C. Anti-HIV Herbs

Azedothymidine, known as AZT, is able to halt reproduction of the AIDS virus. AZT is the only drug approved by the "Food and Drug Administration" (FDA) to fight AIDS. Use of this therapeutic agent is often limited due to its narrow spectrum of antiviral activity and its toxic side effects when administered over long periods (Ruprecht, O'Brien et al, 1986). There is an urgent need to search for less toxic and more effective anti-AIDS virus substances. AIDS virus is more specifically called human immunodeficiency virus (HIV). Chinese herbs appear to be a rich source of potentially useful materials for the treatment of human immunodeficiency virus infection. In fact, Chinese herbs have been used in treatment of AIDS (AIDS Treatment News, 1988). This section will describe the anti-HIV Chinese herbs.

1. Glycyrrhiza radix

Common name: Licorice root
Chinese name: Gan-cao

Licorice is classified as a superior herb in "Shen Nung's Herbal" and is one of the most commonly used herbs in Chinese herbal formulas.

The commonly used licorice roots are the following members of the Leguminosae family: (1) Glycyrrhiza uralensis Fisch. et DC. (2) G. glandulifera WALDSTEIN et KITAIBEL (3) G. echinata L. (4) G. glabra L.

Glycyrrhizine, one of major components of licorece root, has been shown to have an anti-HIV activity (Ito, Nakashima et al, 1987). The combination of glycyrrhizin with AZT resulted in an additive inhibitory effect on HIV, suggesting that glycyrrhizin and AZT attack HIV in different ways.

2. Hypericum

Common name: Saint John's wort
Chinese name: Tian-Ji-Huang

Hypericum was not recorded in Pen tsao kang mu (Compendium of Chinese Medicinal Herbs) of the Ming Dynasty (1368-1644).

Therefore, hypericum was used as a medicinal herb after the Ming Dynasty.

The Chinese medicinal herbs used in the family Hypericum are Hypericum japonicum, H. perforatum L. and H. erectum THUNB.

Two compounds hypericin and pseudohypericin isolated from Hypericum triquetrifolium Turra have been found to have potent anti-HIV activity (Meruelo, Lavie, and Lavie, 1988). Administration of these compounds to mice at the low doses sufficient to prevent HIV-induced disease appears devoid of undesirable side effects. These compounds have been previously administered to humans as antidepressants (Daniel, 1949). This lack of toxicity at therapeutic doses and availability of hypericum herbs throughout the world enhance the potential of therapeutic use of the herb.

Hypericum perforatum and H. erectum THUNB. are known to contain hypericin (Hsu, Shen et al, 1986). However, cattle and horses develop dermatitis and hair loss after exposure to sunlight after ingestion of these plants.

The following 11 Chinese herbs have been found to have anti-HIV activity from 27 anti-infective Chinese herbs (Chang and Yeung, 1988):

3. Viola Yedoensis

Common name: Viola
Chinese name: Zi-Hua-Ti-Ting

Viola was first recorded in "Compendium of Chinese Medicinal Herbs" (Li Shih-Chen, 1590) in the Ming Dynasty (1368-1644). Traditionally, Viola is used to relieve inflammation.

4. Alternanthera philoxeroides

In Taiwan, Alternanthera sessilis R. Brown ex Roem. & Schultes is used instead of A. philoxeroedes. In Shanghai and Chechiang province in China, hypericum ascyron L is used. Commonly, Eclipta prostrata is used in Chinese herbal formulas.

Common name: Eclipta
Chinese name: Han-Lian-Cao

5. Andrographis paniculata

Common name: Adrographis
Chinese name: Chuan-Xin-Lian

Andrographis is not recorded in any traditionsl Chinese herbal books. Andrographis paniculata belongs to Acanthaceae family. Traditionally, this herb is used for tonsillitis, bronchitis, pneumonia, acute enteritis, urethritis, ncphritis,and pustular dermatitis.

6. Arctium lappa L.

Common name: Burdock
Chinese name: Niu-Bang-Zi

Arctium lappa is listed in Ming yi pieh lu (A collection of Famous Prescriptions, A.D. 500) as a general herb drug. The herb was introduced into China from Europe in ancient times. Arctium lappa belongs to Compositae family.

Traditionally, it is used for the common cold, coughs, sore throat, the unerupted erythema, and carbuncles.

7. Lithospermum erythrorhizon

Common name: Purple Gromwell Root
Chinese name: Zi-Cao

Lithospermum is recorded in "Shen Nung's Herbal" as a general herb drug. It belongs to the Borginaceae family. Traditionally, the herb is used for macula, tumor, swelling and constipation.

8. Coptis Chinensis

Common name: Coptis
Chinese name: Huang-Lien

Coptis is listed in "Shen Nung's Herbal" as a superior herb drug. Various species are sold in the market. Coptis chinensis Franch is mostly produced in Szechuan province and C. teetoides C.Y. Cheng is the product of Yunnan province in China. C. japonica grows mostly in Japan. They are the members of the Ranunculaceae family.

Traditionally, coptis is used for edema, fever and thirst, diarrhea due to heat, abdominal pain, hemoptysis, epistaxis and conjunctivitis.

9. Epimedium grandiflorum

Common name: Epimedium
Chinese name: Yin-Yang-Huo

Epimedium is listed in Shen Nung's herbal as a general herb drug. The Chinese name, Yin-Yang-Huo is derived from northern Szechuan province where it is believed that the animal Yin-Yang takes this herb, huo, to stimulate his sexual climax every day. Epimedium belongs to the Berberidaceae family. E. asgittatum (Sieb. et Zucc) MAXIM is commonly used in Chinese herbal medicine. E. sagittatum MAXIM and E. sinense SIEB are same herb.

Traditionally, it is used for impotence, general paralysis, and weakness in the loins and knees.

The herb extract has been found to have hypotensive, antitussive, expectorant, and antiasthmatic effects (Kiangsu New Medical College, 1978). The root and rhizome contain vitamin E.

10. Lonicera japonica

a. Lonicerae Caulis et Folium

Common name: honeysuckle stem
Chinese name: Jen-Tong-Teng also called Yin-hua-teng

Lonicera is recorded in Tang pen tsao (Tang's Herbal) and Chien Chin i fang (Precious Herbal Formulas) in the Tang Dynasty (618- 907). L. japonica belongs to the Caprifoliaceae family. The dried stem and leaf are used in Chinese herbal medicine.

Traditionally, it is used for arthralgia.

b. Lonicerae Flos

Common name: Honeysuckle
Chinese name: Iin-Yin-Hua

The dried flower bud of L. japonica is used in Chinese herbal medicine. It is first recorded in "A Collection of Famous Presecip-tions" as a superior herb drug by the name of Jen-tong. It was later listed as Jin-Yin-Hua in the "Compendium of Chinese Medicinal Herbs" due to the fact the white flower turns from silver to golden in color as it matures.

Traditionally, it is used for carbuncle, fever, dermal eruptions and malignant ulcers.

11. Prunella vulgaris

Common name: Prunella
Chinese name: Xia-Ku-Cao

Prunella was first recorded in the "Compendium of Chinese Medicinal Herbs" as an inferior herb drug. The Chinese name, Xia-Ku-Cao, means that the herb withers after summer because of its nature. Prunella belongs to the Labiatae family.

Traditionally, it is used for conjunctivitis, ocular swelling and pain, photophobia, goiter and scrofula.

12. Senecio scandens

Common name: Senecio
Chinese name: Qian-Li-Guang

Senecio is recorded in Pen tsao shih yi (A Compilation of Chinese Medicinel Herbs, A.D. 739) and Tu ching pen tsao (Chinese Herbal with Illustration, A.D. 1061). It is believed that the herb can brighten the eye to see through a "thousand miles." Qian-li means a thousand miles and Guang means light. S. Acan-dens belongs to the compositae family.

Traditionally, it is used for acute inflammatory diseases, nebula, hyperemia of the eye, septicemia and dysentery due to intestinal inflammation.

13. Woodwardia unigemmata

In Chinese Materia Medica, Woodwardia is listed with Cibotii Rhizoma. Woodwardia orientalis SW (Blechnaceae family) and Cibotium barometz (L.) Smith (Duksoniaceae family) are commonly used in Chinese herbal medicine instead of W. unigemmata. Therefore, Chinese herb Gou-Ji means either C. barometz or woodwardia.

Gou-ji is listed in "Shen Nung's Herbal" as a general herb drug.

Traditionally, it is used for foot and knee debility, knee pain, waist and back pain and enuresis.

D. Clinical Reports

Report 1.

A 38-year-old Caucasian AIDS patient was treated by Dr. Keji Chen, visiting professor from the China Academy of Traditional Chinese Medicine and Director of Beijing Xiyuan Hospital, and Dr. Jean Yu of the Santa Barbara College of Oriental Medicine, California.

The patient was diagnosed HIV positive in May, 1984. The patient complained of chronic diarrhea, depression, and swollen non-tender lymphnodes for 3 to 4 years. The findings on the physical examination were unremarkable except for the symptoms of the lymphoreticular system. The patient had non-streptococcal pharyngitis and his lymph nodes were found to be enlarged 3x4x2cm in the auxillary, inguinal and posterior cervical areas. Splenic enlargement was detected by palpation. Laboratory tests found that serum glutamic-oxaloacetic transaminase (SGOT) and serum glutamic-pyruvic transaminase (SGPT) were abnormally high with 136 IU/L and 268 IU/L respectively. Prothrombin time was 15.2 sec in comparison to a normal value of 11 to 13 sec. Candidas were found on the tongue by culture tests.

Tongue pictures showed red and delicate bodies with a longitudinal crack; the tip and edge had red spots, a thin yellowish greasy coating and thickness towards the root. Pulse showed rapid (over 90/min), wiry and slippery. According to "Traditional Chinese Medicine diagnosis," the patient was diagnosed as having warm-toxic-symptom-complex located in both Chi and blood with deficiencies in his kidney, spleen, and heart.

Table. 18 Detoxifying Formula

Herb	Immunological Activity
Aesculi wilsonii	Anti-inflammatory
Baphicacanthes cusia	Anti-bacterial,anti-inflammatory
Crataegus cuneata	Anti-bacterial
Forsythia suspensa	Anti-bacterial, antiviral
Hordeum vulgare	Interferon inducer
Isatis tinctoria	Anti-bacterial, antiviral
Lonicera japonica	Anti-HIV
Oldenlandia diffusa	Immunostimulating polysaccharides
Paeonia lactiflora	Interferon inducer
Scutellaria baicalensis	Interferon inducer

The Chinese herbal treatment was set for three stages. The first stage used the modified Ganlu Xiaodu Yin (Detoxifying formula) for clearing heat, cooling blood, eliminating dampness and toxic factors (May 1986-August, 1986). The second stage used the modified Shenmai San (Tonifying formula) to tonify Chi and Yin

(October, 1986-March, 1987) and the third stage used Ginseng and Longan combination with double or triple amount of Astragalus membranaceus in the formula to vitalize the body and tonify the kidneys (May, 1987- September, 1987). After a 17-month treatment, the diarrhea was gone. The sore throat was no longer a main complaint and shrinkage of adenopathy was observed. SGOT and SGPT values were reduced to 73 IU/L and 169 IU/L, respectively. The patient's subjective feeling was much improved. The patient has started to work in a part-time job and attend a vocational school.

Table 19. Tonifying Formula

Herb	Immunological Activity
Alternanthera philoxeroides	Anti-HIV
Ligustrum lucidum	Anti-cancer
Ophiopogin japonicus	Anti-bacterial,anti-inflammatory
Panax ginseng	Immunostimulating polysacchorides Interferon inducer
Schizandra Chinensis	Interferon inducer

Tsung's Analysis

The formulas used in the treatment were analysed by the scientific basis so far documented in scientific journals. Table 18, 19, and 20 show the analysis. The first stage treatment focused on the suppression of HIV, other viral infection and anti-bacterial infection.

It is well known now that many bacterial infections and certain tumors, paticularly Kaposis' sarcoma of the skin and certain lymphomas, have become the defining features of AIDS. The interferon-inducing herbs also enhance the activity to fight virus infections and tumors. Finally, the immunostimulating herb, Oldenladia diffusa, can strengthen the body's immune system.

Table 20. Ginseng and Longan Combination plus

Herb	Immunological activity
Angelica Ainansis	Immunostimulating polysaccharides Interferon inducer
Astragalus membranaceus	Immunostimulating polysaccharides Interferon inducer
Atractylodes ovata	Interferon inducer
Euphoria longana	Anti-bacterial
Glycyrrhiza uralensis	Anti-HIV, Interferon inducer
Panax ginseng	Immunostimulating polysaccharides Interferon inducer
Polygala tenuifolia	Interferonn inducer, anti-bacterial
Poria cocos	Immunostimulating polysaccharides
Saussurea lappa	Anti-bacterial
Zingiber officinale	Interferon inducer, anti-bacterial
Zizyphus jujuba (fruit)	Anti-allergic, cAMP
Zizyphus jujuba (seed)	cAMP

In the second stage, the Tonifying formula contains 4 tonic herbs in addition to anti-HIV. The Four tonic herbs are ligustrum, ophiopogon, ginseng and schizandra. The anti-cancer, anti-bacterial, interferon-inducing and immunostmulating properties of the herbs allow the body to fight HIV and AIDS associated infections with tonifying herbal functions.

The third formula, Ginseng and Longan Combination plus, emphasizes the activation of the body's immune system by using 4 immunostimulating polysaccharides containing herbs as shown in

Table 20. The anti-HIV herb used in the formula was Glycyrrhiza uralensis. Cyilic AMP containing zizyphus fruit and seed, has the anti-allergic function since cyclic AMP is known to have a regulatory effect on allergies (Cyong and Hanabusa, 1980; Hanabusa et al, 1981). Seven out of 12 herbs in the formula have interferon-inducing activity and four herbs have anti-bacterial activity.

In conclusion, Drs. Yu and Chen used well-balanced herbal formulas for the treatment of AIDS patients.

Report 2

Keith Barton, M.D., C.A., a California physician, has been using the anti-HIV Chinese herbal combination to treat AIDS patients in Berkeley, California.

He has been treating AIDS patients with a herbal combination of Viola, Lithesperma, Lonicera flos, Prunella, Epimedium, and Licorice. All six herbs have the anti-HIV activity as mentioned in the previous section. He is also using a different herbal combination called Isatis 6 which contains isatis, viola, prunella, taraxacum, and andrographis. Andrographis, Prunella, and Viola have anti-HIV activity and Isatis has antibacterial and antiviral activities (Namba, 1980; Takagi et al, 1982). Taraxacum has antibacterial and antifungal activities (Kiangsu New Medical college, 1978; Namba,1980; Takagi et al, 1982).

He has been using HIV p24 antigen level, total white cells count, T-lymphocyte count, and beta-2 microglobulin in serum as his markers for the evaluation of the Chinese herbal therapy.

For more information send a self-addressed stamped envelope to:

Keith Barton, M.D., 3099 Telegraph Avenue, Barkeley, CA 94705.

It is of importance to know whether adding interferon-inducing and immunostimulating herbs to Dr. Barton's all anti-HIV 6 herbal combinution can accelerate the improvement of AIDS patient conditions.

Report 3

The Lincoln Hospital Acupuncture Clinic in New York City has been using acupuncture and Chinese herbs to treat people with AIDS and AIDS-Related Complex (ARC) since 1982. Lincoln Hospital also has prepared a protocol for a controlled research evaluation of the effects of the combination of acupuncture and Chinese herbs in AIDS treatment. Dr. Angela Shen has been supervising this particular project with promising results.

Preliminary results at Lincoln Hospital indicate that the addition of Chinese herbs in AIDS treatment has obtained remarkable results (Smith, 1987). They are planning a clinical trial of one to two year's duration so that more definite results can be obtained. Also, they reported a reduction of chemotherapy side effects with Chinese medical treatment. Inquiries concerning this program may be addressed to : Dr. Michael O. Smith, Lincoln Hospital. Acupuncture Clinic, 349 East 140th Street, Bronx, NY 10454.

Report 4

The Somerville Acupuncture Center near Boston has treated AIDS and ARC patients with acupuncture and Chinese herbs. Their Chinese herbal treatment focuses on gentle tonification of Yin and blood.

Report 5

A more intensive Chinese herbal program for AIDS treatment has been developed by the Quan Yin Acupuncture Clinic in San Francisco with the collaboration of the Oriental Healing Arts Institute. Their objective is to provide HIV(+) people with a consistent herbal therapy program and to maintain records of the treatments used and the progress of each person. The herbal therapy principles are based on detoxification (Westen medicinal term: anti-inflammatory, antiviral, antibacterial treatments) and immune-enhancement. The theoretical basis is identical to what Drs. Yu and Chen used in their herbal therapy in Report 1.

After the six-month program, they have concluded that the formulas they used generally made people feel better, helped them to fight certain infections better, and seemed to raise red blood cell levels. However, adding herbs which can stimulate bone marrow cells to produce T-lymphocytes and white blood cells is necessary to fight anemia and to increase white blood cell counts (Cohen, 1989).

E. Other Retroviruses Found Spreading Among Drug Users in the United States

Human T-cell leukemia virus type I (HTLV-I), HTLV-II and the AIDS virus are members of a class of retrovirus that were not known to infect humans until recently.

According to new surveys, HTLV-II has been found in about 20 percent of a group of drug addicts in New Orleans, 4 to 10 percent of a group of drug users in New York, and 20 percent of a group of New York drug addicts who were also suffering from AIDS. Like the AIDS virus, HTLV-II is thought to be spread through blood, sexual intercourse and shared needles.

Dr. David Golde of the University of California, Los Angeles, discovered HTLV-II in 1982 in collaboration with Dr. Robert C. Gallo of the National Cancer Institute. HTLV-II was originally isolated from patients with an unusual leukemia called hairy-cell lenkemia. A young man living in California was the first discovered patient of HTLV-II infection in the United States.

A preliminary survey of blood donors in San Francisco area found that HTLV-II, though very rare, was more widespread than the AIDS virus. Another survey reported that HTLV-II is more prevalent in blood donors in Los Angeles and New Orleans than San Francisco. HTLV-II does not appear to pose a significant threat to the nation's blood supply because blood banks have recently instituted a screening test to eliminate the AIDS related virus, including, HTLV-II.

HTLV-II is closely related to another virus, HTLV-I, which causes leukemia and a progressive neurological disorder similar to multiple sclerosis. Researchers do not know at the moment whether HTLV-II also causes hairy-cell leukemia. However, HTLV-II converts normal white blood cells to leukamia cells in laboratory experiments.

HTLV-I is endemic in Japan and the Caribbean. It usually takes 10 to 20 years for people infected with HTLV-I to develop leukemia and neurological disorders. Experts estimate that 1 to 2 percent of people infected with the virus eventrally become ill.

In animals, retroviruses cause cancer.

F. Concluding Remarks

Various practitioners have been applying Chinese herbal medicine to treat AIDS patients since the begining of the AIDS epidemic. However, the application of Chinese herbal medicine to AIDS patients has not intensified until the past two to three years. This is largely due to the finding of anti-AIDS virus activity in various Chinese herbs in addition to immunostimulating activity. The side effects and shortage of AZT also accelerate the usage of Chinese herbal medicine because of its low cost and non-detectable side effects. In addition, new studies show the AIDS virus is becoming resistant to AZT. The use of Chinese herbal medicine will be much in demand from now on.

Many hospitals, acupuncture clinics and private practitioners have organized their Chinese herbal treatment projects on their AIDS patients nationwide. More Western-trained physicians are participating in the projects with acupuncturists and Chinese herbalists. As mentioned in the clinical reports, the results are very encouraging and promising.

In the effort to expand herbal treatment projects, all of us involved in Chinese herbal medicine programs should campaign hard to get funds from the Federal goverment, State, and other financial sources to overcome the deadly disease.

The present health and social services system is unable to deal with the diverse needs of people who are HIV positive. The services are uncoordinated and fragmented. People who are HIV positive but without symptoms should take anti-HIV and immunostimulating herbs as early as possible to suppress the AIDS virus. Premininary results in the herbal treatment indicate that the successful rate of suppression of the AIDS virus is higher when the patient's HIV antigen level is still at low.

It has been shown that Chinese herbal formulas can reduce the side effect of chemotherapy in AIDS patients (Smith, 1987). Therefore, it would be worthwhile to expand the herbal treatment with AZT or other chemotherapies.

Areas of effort should include basic biological research on Chinese herbs and Chinese herbal formulas.

IX
Hepatitis and
Chinese Herbs

A. Introduction

It was reported at the conference on Acquired Immune Deficiency Syndrome and hepatitis B that hepatitis, a viral-liver disease, is spreading in the same manner as AIDS in the United States.

Hepatitis is a viral disease that attacks the liver, causing jaundice, fatigue and loss of appetite. Hepatitis A is spread mostly through food and is generally a mild disease. However, hepatitis B is spread through an exchange of bodily fluids, usually through sexual contact or from mother to child during birth. The sharing of drug needles also transfers the virus. Hepatitis B is thought to be the major cause of primary liver cancer and is thought to cause about 5,000 deaths a year, either directly or indirectly, in the United States, according to the National Foundation for Infectious Diseases.

Hepatitis B has a long incubation period of several months but the serious effects of the disease, such as cancer or liver failure, might not appear for decades in chronic carriers.

There is a vaccine against hepatitis B. The vaccine can prevent the disease, but it cannot cure it once a patient is infected. And the vaccine is expensive. It costs about $120 for the recommended three-shot series.

The number of U.S. hepatitis B cases has increased from 200,000 in 1978 to about 300,000 in 1988. On a global basis, the problem is even more severe. There are an estimated 300 million cases worldwide.

B. Clinical reports

Advances in medical and pharmaceutical sciences have enabled us to gain control over many contagious diseases. However, viral hepatitis has no medicine to cure the disease. In Western medicine, liver diseases are considered difficult to treat effectively. A large number of Chinese herbal formulas, however, are believed to be effective on hepatitis.

Report 1

Minor Bupleurum Combination (MBC) has long been used to treat hepatitis. The original sources and ingredients have been described in Chapter IV. Briefly, the functions of each herb in the ingredients are summarized in Table 21.

Table 21. The functions of each herb in MBC

Bupleurum	Anti-inflammatory, interferon-inducing
Ginger	Anti-Oxidant, interferon-inducing
Ginseng	Immunostimulating, interferon-inducing
Jujube	Anti-allergic
Liorice	Anti-viral, interferon-inducing
Pinellia	Interferon-inducing
Scute	Antiviral, interferon-inducing

Shigeru Arichi of Kinki University, Japan, treated 26 hepatitis B patients with MBC. Seventy-seven percent of the patients showed great improvement in both subjective and objective symptoms within 8 weeks after receiving MBC treatment (Arichi, 1978; Arichi and Tani, 1980; Arichi, 1981). The level of hepatitis marker enzymes, glutamic oxaloacetic transaminase (GOT) and glutamic pyruric transaminase (GPT) had returned to normal following treatment with MBC.

As shown in Table 21, MBC contains antiviral, anti-allergic, anti-inflammatory, anti-oxident, immunostimulating, and interferon-inducing activities.

Report 2

Qe-wang Jin and Associates of the Wusung City Infectious Diseases Hospital treated 50 hepatitis B patients with immunostimulating and interferon-inducing herbs with promising results. The immunostimulating and interferon-inducing herbs are Astragalus membranaceus, Olderlandia diffusa, Schizandra chinensis, and Scutellaria baicalensis. In addition, they used Salvia milliorrhiza to enhance blood circulation.

The level of hepatitis marker enzyme returned to normal in 46% of patients and 6% of patients showed negative levels in hepatitis B antigen in serum after 12 weeks of treatment. Forty percent of patients resulted in 4-fold decrease of hepatitis B antigen levels after treatment.

Report 3

Shuchang Yan and Associates of the China Academy of Traditional Chinese Medicine treated 538 patients of chronic viral hepatitis for 5 years with immunostimulating polysaccharide isolated from Polyporus umbellatus (Yan, 1988). About 39% of the patients became negative in hepatitis antigen in their serum and 38% of the patients decreased more than 4-fold in their hepatitis antigen levels after treatment.

The serum GPT level returned to normal in 36% of the patients and 42% of the patients decreased their GPT levels more than 50% after treatment.

The efficacy of the polysaccharide therapy was examined in a 2-4 year follow-up of patients and the results were positive and stable.

They treated the patients by injection. It is important to know whether oral administration of the polysaccharide would be effective treatment.

Report 4

Obata, et al (1984) treated 25 hepatitis antigen positive patients with glycyrrhizin (aquequs extract of licorice root) for 8 weeks and found that 14 patients became hepatitis antigen negative during a follow-up period of 6 months to 1 year. The immunological activities of glycyrrhizin were described in previous chapters.

Report 5

In Japan, cardiac surgery clinics administer glycyrrhizin to all hospitalized persons to prevent the spread of hepatitis. The prevention trial of post-transfusion hepatitis in surgical clinics with glycyrrhizin was first conducted by Sekiguchi, et al, (1982).

C. Concluding Remarks

Since we know now that many Chinese herbs are effective in treating and preventing hepatitis, we can use these herbs as dietary supplements in our daily life. This not only can prevent hepatitis but also can enhance our immune system to prevent other diseases, too.

The administration of licorice root extract glycyrrhizin, in the prevention of post-transfusion and post-surgery hepatitis can also apply in prevention of the AIDS virus infection since glycyrrhizin is also known to have anti-HIV activity. Its administration is now a routine practice in hospitals in Japan. Therefore, there is no reason that we cannot administer it here in the United States.

X
Diabetes and Chinese Herbs

A. Introduction

Insulin-dependent diabetes affects more than a half million individuals in the United States. Over the past few years, researchers have come to a growing acceptance of the hypothesis that insulin-dependent diabetes is caused by an autoimmune attack that destroys the insulin-producing beta cells of the pancreas.

What causes the initial beta cell damage is still uncertain. Viral infections and toxic chemicals have both been proposed as initiating agents. And interleukin-1, a substance released from macrophage, has also been proposed (Mandrup-Poulsen, 1987).

All diabetes are not insulin-dependent. An additional 9 to 10 million people have non-insulin-independent diabetes, which usually develops later in life and is apparently a different disease.

Chinese herbal formulas have been used in the treatment of diabetes in China, Japan, and many other Asian countries for more than two thousand years. The most commonly used 2 formulas will be discussed in the following section.

B. Commonly Used Chinese Herbal Formulas

1. Ginseng and Gypsum Combination

Ingredients: Anemarrhena, Ginseng, Gypsum, Licorice, Oryza.

Ginseng and Gypsum Combination was recorded in both the "Treatise on Febrile Diseases" and "Prescriptions from the Golden Chamber" by Chang Chung-Ching during the Han Dynasty (207 B.C.-220 A.D.).

Immunologically active polysaccharide has been isolated from ginseng (Mizutani, Ohtani et al, 1985). It has been shown that the polysaccharide possesses both active site and inhibitory site in the polysaccharide structure (Kiyohara, et al, 1985; Nagai, et al, 1985). It is therefore suggested that the polysaccharide modulates the immune system depending on body conditions. The concept of "adaptogen" is born due to ginseng's regulatory activity. It is reasonable to assume that ginseng in the formula might act as an immunomodulator to reduce the autoimmune attack on beta cells of the pancreas.

Licorice is known to have antiviral activity. Under the hypothesis that viral infection causes the initial beta cell damage, then licorice in the ingredients coincides with the hypothesis to eliminate the viral infection.

Anemarrhena was first recorded in "Shen Nung's Herbal." The medicinal part is the dried rhizome of Anemarrhana asphodeloides BUNGE. Blood sugar-reducing activity has been shown in the aqueous extract (Kimura, 1967; Kohda, et al, 1971; Takagi, 1982). Recently, a polysaccharide anemaren C has been isolated from the herb. The anemaran C also shows the blood sugar-reducing activity (Takahashi et al, 1985).

Oryza is the peeled seed of oryza sativa L of the Gramineae family. Oryza is rich in vitamin B1 and enzymes such as phytase, lipase and diastase.

Gypsum is considered a sedative which dispels heat in Chinese medicine concepts. Since calcium has been considered to have cellular regulatory function, I will considered gypsum as a calcium source.

2. Rehmannia Eight Formula

Ingredients: rehmannia, Cinnamon, aconite, hoelen, dioscorea, alisma, moutan, cornus

The functions of each herb are summarized in Table 22.

Table 22. The functions of each herb in Rehmannia Eight Formula

Herb	Function
Aconite	Anti-inflammatory
Alisma	Reduces blood sugar
Cinnamon	Anti-allergic
Cornus	Anti-allergic
Dioscorea	Interferon-inducing
Hoelen	Immunologicallyactive polysaccharide
Moutan	Anti-allergic
Rehmannia	Interferon-inducing

As shown in Table 22, 7 out of 8 herbs in the formula are related to the immune system. The combination of the immunomodulating 7 herbs in some way and somehow might be able to reduce the autoimmune attack on the insulin-producing beta cells of the pancreas. Alisma can lower the blood sugar level to help the regulation of sugar metabolism.

Rehmannia Eight Formula has been used as an anti-cataract drug in Japan (Fujihira, 1973). Cataracts, which cloud the lenses of the eyes, are a major health problem, resulting in more than 1 million operations in the United States each year to correct the problem. Senile cataracts have been a significant problem of blindness for diabetic patients or elderly people. Kinoshita, et al (Kinoshita, 1974; Varma and Kinoshita, 1974) have reported that the mechanism of diabetic cataract is due to accumulation of polyol, which was reduced from sugar by aldose reductase in the lens. From animal experiments, it has been suggested that Rehmannia Eight formula may have a prophylactic effect on diabetic cataracts (Kamei, Hisada and Iwata, 1987).

C. Concluding Remarks

It has been hypothesized that diabetes is an autoimmune disease. Two commonly used Chinese herbal formulas have been discussed along with their immunological activities. The prophylactic effect of Rehmannia Eight Formula on diabetic cataracts has been suggested by biochemical analysis in animal experiments. The advance in modern technologies enables us to solve the puzzles one by one in Chinese herbal medicine.

XI
Enhance Children's Immunity with Chinese Herbs

A. Introduction

Most pediatricians will say that most children have had a hundred upper respiratory infections by the time they are 10 years old. Certainly runny noses, sore throats, coughs and earaches are most common symptoms in most sick children seen in pediatrician's offices.

The treatment of upper respiratory infections hasn't really changed much in the last 25 years. Most children with colds would get better with remedies their grandparents used. There is no Western medicine for the common cold anyway.

Children are born with very little immunity. They have received from their mothers some antibodies. But most of these antibodies disappear during the first year of life. An antibody is an immunoglobulin molecule that combats each infection specifically. In the process of acquiring immunity, the infection itself is the step that makes its own specific antibodies for that specific infections. However, some children are frequently getting sick and some children are much quicker than others to recover from infection. Immunity build-up in each child might be different due to genetic, nutritional and unknown factors as well as the mother's immunological condition.

Some groups of children who get sick more often than other children are called "kyojaku-ji" (weak child) in Japan. For these kinds of children, Japanese pediatricians are prescribing Chinese herbal formulas to enhance their immunities. Of course the Chinese have been doing this for more than three thousand years. The commonly used prescriptions on such children will be discussed in the following section.

B. Immunostimulating Herbal Formulas for Frequently Sick Children

1. Dr. Hirose's report

Dr. S. Hirose is head of the Pediatric Department in Kariya Hospital in Japan. His pediatric department treats more than 100 patients a day. More than 50% of the patients are freqrent visitors of the department. Their symptoms include fever, common cold, fatigue and respiratory infections. For these "Kyojaku-ji", he prescribes Astragalus Combination and Minor Bupleurum Combination with remarkable success (Hirose, 1989). He also prescribes these herbal formulas to treat his own children.

Astragalus Combination contains astragalus, cinnamon, ginger, jujube, licorice, maltose, and peony. As mentioned in the previous chapters, astragalus possesses immunostimulating polysaccharides and interferon-inducing activity and licorice has antiviral and interferon-inducing activities. Cinnamon, ginger and jujube have anti-allergic activity. And anti-bacterial and antiviral activities have been found in peony. Minor Bupleurum Combination has been described so many times in the previous Chapters as an immunostinulating formula, the detailed description will not be mentioned here.

2. Tsung's formula

My son catches cold very often and is always coughing, sneezing and suffering from a runny nose. Since taking Minor Blue Dragon Combination and Coptis & Scute Combination, his symptoms have gone.

Minor Blue Dragon Combination is an excellent formula for rhinitis and Coptis & Scute Combination possesses herbs of anti-bacterial, anti-fungal, anti-viral, anti-inflammatory, and antipyretic activities. Minor Blue Dragon Combination contains pinellia, peony, cinnamon, schizandra, Ma-huang, licorice, asarum and ginger. Coptis & Scute combination contains coptiss, scute, gardenia, and phellodendron.

3. Traditional Chinese formulas

Traditionally, most Chinese families serve a tonic soup to their children in the winter time. The popular tonic herbs are ginseng, Tang-kuei (Angelica) and astragalus, and most commonly used herbal combinations are Ginseng and Ginger Combination, Ginseng and Astragalus Combination, and Ginseng and Tang-kuei Ten Conbination. The tonic herbs or the tonic herbal combination are served either as tea or incorporated in chicken soup, fish soup or meat soup. These tonic herbs or tonic herbal combinations are known to have immunostimulating functions. Winter usually is the common cold season. This is the reason that the tonic tea or soup is served in winter.

C. Concluding Remarks

The traditional Chinese way to enhance children's immunities by tonic herbs turns out to be very scientific due to the herbs possessing immunostimulating, interferon-inducing, antiviral, antibacterial, antifugal, antiallergic and anti-inflammatory activities.

Many Japanese pediatricians have used the immunostimulating Chinese herbal formulas with great success on their patients who are frequently getting respiratory infections. Minor Blue Dragon Combination has been used to treat allergic rhinitis in adults as well as children with remarkable results in China and Japan.

This chapter does not intend to advocate minimal medical care for children. Periodic checkups are important and immunization is a must. Many childhood diseases are completely preventable. Furthermore, a basic understanding of the mechanism of an illness that may occur can help a parent initiate home remedies that work.

XII
Radiation Protection effect of Chinese Herbs

A. Introduction

It is well known that above a certain level, radiation causes damage of the immune system in the body. The result of the aftermath of Hiroshima and Nagasaki is a good example. A large dose of radiation results in immediate risk of death and longer term risk of chronic tissue damage. It also causes mutations in the cells. Leukemia was about 100 times more common in Japanese Atombomb survivors than in non-exposed Japanese. Much controversy has been aroused on the question of the possible harmful effects of diagnostic X-rays, and a great many pages both for and against the idea that X-rays can cause harm have been written.

Since we do know that radiation damages bone marrow cells that produce the immune cells and blood cells, some thought has been given to the question of whether all workers involved with nuclear reactors and other people at special risk of accidental radiation exposure should have some of their bone marrow cells stored away in case of a disaster. A research group at the Radiation Center of Osaka, Japan, has found that ginseng extract and three Chinese herbal formulas have radiation protection effect (Yonezawa, Hosokawa et al, 1987). Their report is deseribed in the following section.

B. Report

There are few radiation-protective substances of low toxicity practically applicable to man that restore serious damage to the blood-forming tissues through post-irradiation. Since ginseng is known as a hemopoiesis stimulant (Yamamoto, Masada et al, 1977), the radiation-protective effect of ginseng was tested in experimental animals in comparison with three other Chinese herbal formulas.

When mice were irradiated with 720 roentgen (R) of X-ray, they died from 10 to 20 days after the irradiation. Injection of 1.8mg of ginseng extract to the mice within 5 min. after the x-ray irradiation increased survival rates 45% and injection of 6.8mg of ginseng extract increased the percentage survival to about 83%. Similar results were obtained in rat and guinea pig experiments. Ginseng enhanced the recovery of blood forming stem cells in bone marrow of irradiated mice (Yonezawa, Katoh and Takeda, 1985).

The oral administration of Chinese herbal formulas (Minor Bupleurum Combination, Ginseng and Astragalus Combination, Ginseng and Tang-kuei Ten Conbination) prior to irradiation obtained the same results. Acanthopanax senticosus also has radiation-protective activity (Yonezawa, Katoh, and Takeda, 1981a).

The radiation-protective principle(s) is not ginseng saponins (Yonezawa, Katoh and Tadeda, 1981b), and the primary results indicate that the radiation-protective principle is some kind of glycopeptide or peptidoglycan.

C. Concluding Remarks

Since ginseng and three Chinese herbal formulas have rediation-protective activity, the application of ginseng or the herbal formulas to cancer radiotherapy will be very beneficial to cancer patients.

In addition, radiation department workers in hospitals, diagnostic x-rays technicians in dental offices, all workers involved with nuclear reactors, and other people at special risk of accidental radiation exposure are recommended to take ginseng or the other three herbal formulas as a diet supplement for their protection.

XIII
Old Concept,
New Idea

Why are Chinese herbal medicines always the combination of more than two herbs? Since it has been this way for more than three thousand years, it must have reasons. I have been searching for the answer for a long time. The following are the answers that I found in scientific documents.

1. Some components in the formula can promote the solubility and absorption of the herbs' pharmacologically active components

Research of the pharmacological and physiological activities of components separated from various Chinese herbs and Chinese herbal formulas has been widely developed in recent years and scientific explanations for the effectiveness of many herbal formulas have emerged. However, activities discovered in crude extracts tend to decrease or disappear when such extracts are purified. Moreover, water-soluble components in the crude extracts tend to become insoluble as the components are purified.

It is reasonable to assume that there must be other components which are capable of increasing the water solubility of the active components and promoting their absorption in the digestive tract in addition to the herbs' pharmacologically and physiologically active components. The effectiveness of the Chinese herbal formula is probaly due to the joint action of these substances. The following evidence verifies this hypothesis.

It has been found that ginseng saponins can promote the dissolution of bupleurum saponins (Yata and Tanaka, 1988). Bupleurum saponin a and d are the active components of bupleurum. The purified bupleurum saponin a and d are very difficult to dissolve in water. However, ginseng saponins can markedly increase the solubility of bupleurum saponins. To be effective, in preparation of bupleurum-containing formulas, the extraction has to mix whole herbs with bupleurum together according to the ancient classics of Chinese herbal medicine.

The efficacy of a drug or medicine depends on the absorbability in the digestive tract when administered orally. In order to test whether the components in Chinese herbs have absorption-promoting effects, saponins of Sapindus mukorossi were examined with β-lactam type antibiotics and ampicillin, which have poor absorption in the digestive tract. The unabsorbed portion of the drug disturbs the bacteria flora in the intestine causing diarrhea. Therefore, improvement of the drug's absorbability is clinically desirable. Yata and Tanaka (1988) of the Hiroshima University Medical School have been able to show the absorption-promoting effect of sapindus saponins on ampicillin and β-lactam antibiotics by using the in situ loop method on the small intestine and rectum of the mouse.

The above-mentioned evidence verifies the principle of Chinese herbal medicine that the combination of more than two herbs not only enhances the additive effect of all active components but also increases the other aspects of therapeutical effects.

2. The efficacy of each Chinese herbal formula depends on the ratio of the active components

This is entirely my speculation. Since we know from the previous chapters that a formula consists of different herbal combinations depending on the use of the formula, they not only compensate each other pharmacologically but also help each other with therapeutical functions such as absorbability and solubility of the active components. It has been shown that the active site and inhibitory site of an immunomodulating polysaccharide are co-existing in the polysaccharide structure (Kiyohara, et al, 1985; Nagai, et al, 1985). Depending on the herbal combination, the polysaccharide might act either as immunostimulator or immunosuppressor. Tomimori and Yoshimoto (1980) have demonstrated that the extractability of glycyrrhizin, an active component of licorice, depends on the combination of the other herbs.

Therefore, the concentrations of active components regulate each other in the formula and I guess it is essential for the maximum therapeutical effect and optimal function for the formula.

3. Elimination of side effects

Harringtonine and homoharringtonine, compounds isolated from Cephalotaxus fortunei, have been known to be effective against acute chronic granulocytic and monocytic leukemia (Lou and Chen, 1978). However, these have severe toxicity that cause damage to the heart and hematopoietic organs. When anethole, oleanolic acid, and ginsenoside are added to harringtonine and homoharringtonine, the side effects of harringtonine and homoharringtonine are eliminated without effecting the antileukemia activity (U. S. patent 4675318, 1987). Anethole was isolated from Forniculum vulgare and oleanolic acid was isolated from the fruits of ligustrum lucidum. Ginsenoside was iolated from ginseng.

Therefore, even the combination of purified compounds is able to eliminate the side effects or toxicity of chemical compounds.

4. Additive therapeutic effect or activation effect of the combination of two therapeutic drugs

The combination of hypericin or pseudohypericin with azidothymidine (AZT) have been found remarkably effective in curing mice from Friend leukemia virus-induced leukemia at concentrations and frequencies of drug administration in which each of the two drugs separately was ineffective (Meruels, Lavie, and Lavie, 1988). Thus, hypericin and pseudohypericin combined with AZT might improve the therapeutical effect on AIDS.

Hypericin and pseudohypericin have been isolated from the Chinese herb hypericum triquetrifolium (details, see Chapter VII).

5. Eliminate the development of resistance to drugs

The development of bacteria resistant to antibiotics is so common that pharmaceutical companies have to continue to search for new antibiotics. According to a new study, the virus that causes AIDS is becoming resistant to the only FDA approved drug used to treat AIDS, AZT. Chinese herbal formulas have been used for more than three thousand years and we never ever hear bacteria, fungi, and virus becoming resistant to any Chinese herbal formula.

My point in writing this chapter is applying ancient Chinese medical concepts to create new Western medicines cannot only improve therapeutical effects but also can eliminate side effects and development of resistance.

The combination of many compounds and extracts of Chinese herbal combinations would be and should be the future's drug or medicinal concept. I predict it will become a new trend in the pharmaceutical industry soon.

XIV
Conclusion

According to the report entitled "Health, United States, 1988" prepared by the National Center for Health Statistics, U.S. life expectancy rose to a record high of 74.8 years, yet American men die younger than those in Japan, much of Europe, and Cuba, while American women die younger than those in Japan, Canada, Australia and parts of Europe.

The report indicates that the death rate for heart disease declined by 31 percent since 1970, and the rate declined by 53 percent for strokes. The report also says that the dramatic decline in heart disease, strokes and many other conditions is due to the population getting the message on prevention.

Since we know that immunities decline with age and that decreased immunities can result in contraction of diseases, my simple message is to take immunostimulating, interferon-inducing, and antiviral Chinese herbs to boost our immune system against diseases and keep us younger for a happier, healthier life. Antioxidant herbs, tumor necrosis factor-porducing herbs, clearing circulating immune complexes herbs and anti-cataract formula are also good for slowing down the aging process.

In contrast to the aging process, children have to aquire immunity since they are born with very little immunity. Many Chinese herbal formulas can help children to enhance their immunities.

The application of Chinese herbal formulas to AIDS patients has been intensified after the finding of anti-AIDS virus activity in various Chinese herbs in addition to immunostimulating activity. New studies show the AIDS virus is becoming resistant to AZT, the only Food and Drug Administration approved drug. Patients under prolonged use of AZT are not likely to do as well as they do initially. Scientists also said the finding should discourage AZT use among people who are infected with the AIDS virus but not yet ill, because the drug might be fostering resistant strains that would not respond to AZT when such people develop AIDS or AIDS-related complex. The discovery of AZT-resistant virus strains lends increased urgency to develop, test and market alternative AIDS drugs. Since Chinese herbal medicines do not have the side effects of AZT and do not develop resistance, the use of Chinese herbal medicine will be much in demand from now on.

Administration of the licorice root extract, glycyrrhizin has been a routine practice in hospitals in Japan for the prevention of hepatitis in post-transfusion and post-surgery. It will be a nice idea to apply it in the prevention of AIDS virus infection in post-transfusion, since glycyrrhizin has anti-AIDS virus activity.

The Application of X-rays in medical and dental clinics and power supplied by nuclear reactors are examples of our modern technological development, which is increasing our risk of accidental or accumulatory radiation exposure. The radiation-protective Chinese herbs might be able to help workers in these jobs as well as ordinary people.

The combination of more than two herbs has been the concept of Chinese herbal medicine. The tradition has been carried out for more than three thousand years in clinics with millions of patients. The accumulatory wisdom and knowledge formulate the formulas without side effects, eliminating the development of resistance to the formulas, stimulating or regulating the immune system, and with maximum therapeutical effects. Even in Western medicine, the combination of more than two compounds in the drugs will appear in the near future. I predict the combinded use of Chinese herbal medicine with Western medicine will be more popular in clinical use.

The integration of Chinese and Western medicine and medical techniques in the health care and medical system will be very beneficial to our society and all human beings.

[Addendum]

A Protein Isolated From Chinese Herb May Offer Hope For AIDS Victims.

A protein isolated from the Chinese herb Trichosanthes kirilowii has been found to selectively kill human immune system cells that are infected with the AIDS virus. The protein is called trichosanthin, GLQ 223, or Compound Q.

The results were reported in the latest issue of the proceedings of the National Academy of Services. In January 1989, Dr. Michael S. McGrath of San Francisco General Hospital, Dr. Hin-Wing Young of the Chinese University of Hong Kong and two other researchers received U.S. patent 4,795,739 for the use of trichosanthin for AIDS therapies.

The potential breakthrough lies in the fact that trichosanthin not only can interfere with the replication of the AIDS virus, but also can selectively eliminate the virus from key immune system cells, such as T-lymphocytes, monocytes and macrophages, without impairing healthy cells.

The biological and pharmaceutical properties of Trichosanthes kirilowii are described as follows:

    Trichosanthes Radix
    Common Name: Trichosanthes Root
    Chinese Name: Gua-Lou-Gen

Trichosanthes root is recorded in "Chinese Herbal with Illustration," (A.D. 1061) as "Tian-Hua-Fen" (Heaven Flower Powder). The name Heaven Flower Powder is derived from the whitish powder ground the herb's root. Trichosanthes radix is the dried root of Trichosanthes kirilowii MAXIM of the Curcubitaceae family.

Traditionally, this herb is used for the treatment of diabetes, hemorrhoids, jaundice, mastitis, sore throat and swelling.

Pharmacologically, it has blood sugar-lowering and anti-cancer effects. In China, trichosanthes has recently been used to induce abortion.

Trichosanthes seeds, fruit, and rinds also have been used in traditional Chinese herbal medicine. Their properties and actions resemble those of the trichosanthes root.

Reference

McGrath, Michael S., K.M. Hwang, S.E. Caldwell et al.

GLQ223: An inhibitor of human immundeficiency virus replication in acutely and chronically infected cells of lymphocyte and mononuclear phagocyte lineage. Proc. Natl. Acad. Sci. USA vol. 86, pp. 2844-2848, 1989.

Glossary Of Terms

Adrenergic

Activated by, characteristic of, or secreting epinephrine or substances with similar activity.

Alkaloid

One of a large group of organic basic substances found in plants. Examples are atropine, caffeine, morphine, nicotine,quinine.

Antibody

An immunoglobulin molecule that interacts only with the the antigen that induced its synthesis in lymphoid tissue.

Anti-complementary polysaccharide

A polysaccharide which can activate or suppress complement activity.

Antigen

Any substance which is capable of inducing the formation of antibodies and of reacting specifically in some detectable manner with the antibodies so induced.

Basophil

A granular leukocyte which stains readily with basic dyes; one kind of white blood cell.

B-cells

Also called B-lymphocytes. B-cells originate in bone marrow, and are responsible for humoral immunity.

Chemical mediator

Chemical compounds which cause allergic reactions. Histamine, chemotactic factors, and prostaglandin are chemical mediators of all allergic responses.

Ch'i

"Vital essence." This would correspond to the life force, or stock of vitality which must be maintained to ensure health. The idea of ch'i is fundamental to Chinese medical thinking, and no one English word or phrase can adequately capture its meaning.

Complement

The nonspecific factor in fresh serum needed to bring about lysis of a foreign invader. The complement system consists of interacting proteins.

Desensitization

A condition in which the organism does not react immunologically to a specific antigen.

Diuretic

(1) increasing the secretion of urine.
(2) an agent that promotes the secretion of urine.

Endocrine

Secreting internally; applied to organs and structures whose function is to secrete into the blood or lymph a substance (hormone) that has a specific effect on another organ or part.

Ginsenoside

A type of glycoside distributed in ginseng. Glycoside is a compound that contains a carbohydrate molecule con vertible by hydrolytic cleavage into sugar and a nonsugar component. Some glycosides have more than one monosaccharide moiety.

Homeostasis

A tendency toward stability in the normal body states of the organism.

Hypolipemic agent

A substance which can decrease the amount of fat in the blood.

Immunocyte

A cell of the lymphoid series which can react with an antigen to produce antibodies or to become active in cell-mediated immunity.

Immunoglobulin

A protein of animal origin endowed with known antibody activity.

Immunomodulator

An agent which can adjust and/or regulate immune responsiveness.

Immunostimulant

An agent which can stimulate immune responsiveness.

Immunosuppressor

An agent which can suppress immune responsiveness.

Interferon

When viruses of more than one type infect the same cell each may multiply undisturbed by the presence of the others, except for possible recombination or phenotypic mixing. In certain combinations, however, the multiplication of one type of virus may be inhibited to a varying extent, while that of the other types remains normal. This interference can be mediated by a substance produced by virus-infected cells, called interferon.

Leukocytes

White blood cells.

Lymphocyte

An antibody-producing cell.

Lymphokine

A general term for soluble protein mediators thought to be released by sensitized lymphocytes on contact with an antigen, and believed to play a role in macrophage activation, lymphocyte transformation, and cell-mediated immunity.

Lysosome

One of the minute bodies seen with the electron microscope in many types of cells, containing various hydrolytic enzymes and normally involved in the process of localized intracellular digestion.

Macrophage

Any of the large, highly phagocytic cells occurring in the walls of blood vessels and in loose connective tissue. They are components of the reticuloendothelial system. Usually immobile, they become actively mobile when stimulated by inflammation.

Mast Cell

A blood cell which releases histamine upon antigen mediated or antibody-mediated degranulation.

Microbe

A minute form of life capable of causing disease in animals, e.g. bacteria, fungi, and viruses.

Mitogenic

Causing or inducing mitosis, the process by which the body grows and replaces cells.

Monocyte

A mononuclear phagocytic white blood cell.

Mucoregulator

An agent which controls mucus secretion.

Neutrophil

A blood cell. A granular leukocyte having a nucleus with three to five lobes connected by slender threads of chromatin, and cytoplasm containing five inconspicuous granules; called also polymorphonuclear (PMN) leukocyte.

Phagocyte

Any cell that ingests microorganisms or other cells and foreign particles.

Phagocytosis

The engulfing of microorganisms, other cells and foreign particles by phagocytes.

Platelet

A disk-shaped structure found in the blood of all mammals and chiefly known for its rold in blood coagulation.

Polysaccharide

A carbohydrate composd of more than ten saccharide groups.

Reticuloendothelial System

A functional system that serves as an important bodily defense mechanism, composed of highly phagocytic cells having both endothelial and reticular attributes and the ability to take up microorganisms, cell debris, and foreign particles.

Thrombosis

The formaiton, presence, or development of a blood clot.

T-lymphocytes

Two kinds of effector mechanisms mediate immune responses. Antibody-mediated immunity is called humoral immunity. Other immune responses are mediated by cells. The specificity of the cell-mediated immune response depends upon a subset of lymphocytes or T-cells can be divided in subpopulations.

Helper T-cells

T-cells involved in the cytolysis of allogeneic lymphocytes or tumor cells.

Suppressor T-cells

T-cells involved in controlling B-lymphocytes.

Tophi

Plural of tophus. A chalky deposit of urate found in the tissues about the joints in gout.

Yin-Yang Theory

The Theory of Yin and Yang is a life philosophy and a dualistic cosmic theory which explains all activities of the universe, including human life. The universe consists of two basic principles or natures, Yin and Yang; through the change of relationships between these two principles, all creations were formed and are still constantly changing and keeping a state of homeostasis in nature, human societies and individual human beings. The Yang, the male principle, is active and light and is represented by the heavens. The Yin, the female principle, is passive and dark and is represented by the earth. The human body, like matter in general, is made of Yin-Yang. Yin is like a negative electric charge and Yang is a positive electric charge. In the normal condition, the negative charges and positive charges are in neutralized states or in balance. If the balance is disturbed, we are in the condition we call disease.

References

Abe, H., Odashima, S., Konishi H. and Arichi, S. Europ. J. Cell Biol. 22, 390 (1980).

Akabori, A. and Kagawa, S. Shoyakugaku Zasshi,(Japanese Journal of Pharmacognosy) 37, 241 (1983).

Akiyama, Y. and Hamuro, J. Protein, Nucleic Acid and Enzyme, 26, 208 (1981).

Allman, P.L. and Dittner, D.S. eds., The Biolgy Data Book. Federation of American Socities for Experimenal Bioogy, Bethesda, Md. 1972.

Arichi, S. Yakubutsu Ryoho (Chemotherapy) 10, 719 (1978).

Arichi, S. Yakubutsu Ryoho (Chemotherapy) 14, 191 (1981).

Arichi, S. Igaku to Yakugaku,(Medical and Pharmaceutical Science) 8, 415 (1982).

Arichi, S. and Tani, T. Iyaku Journal (Journal of Medicine and Pharmacology) 16, 1285 (1980).

Awad, O. Phytochemistry 13, 678 (1974).

Bansal S.C. and Sjogren, H.O. Int. J. Cancer, 11, 162 (1973).

Bjorksten J. Cross-linkage and the aging process. In: Rockstein M. (ed.) Theoretical Aspects of Aging. New York, Academic Press, p. 43, (1974).

Blackett, A.D. and Hall, D.A., J. Gerontol 36, 529 (1981).

Bomford, R. and Olivotto, M. Int.J. Cancer, 14, 226 (1974).

Bomford, R. and Olivotto, M. C.Parvum: Application to Experimental and Clinical Oncology (ed.B.Halpern),P.270, Plenum Press(1975).

Bradner, W.T.,Clarke, D.A. and Stock, C.C. Cancer Res.,18, 347(1958)

Bradner, W.T. and Clarke, D.A. Cancer Res.,19, 673 (1959).

Brekhman, I.I. and Mayansky G.M. Izv. Akad, Nauk SSSR, Ser. Biol., 5, 762 (1965).

Burnet, F.M. The Clonal Selection Theory of Aquired Immunity. Cambridge, Cambridge University Press (1959).

Chang, Chung-ching, Shang han lun, (Treatise on Febrile Diseases). Han dynasty (219 A.D.). [English translation by Hsu, Hong-Yen and Peacher, William G. (Los Angeles: Oriental Healing Arts Institute,1981).]

Chang, R.S. and Yeung, H.W. Antiviral Research 9, 163-176 (1988).

Chendu Traditional Medical College. Zhong Yao Xue (Chinese Medicine). Shanghai: Science and Technology Press, 1978.

Chihara, G., et al. Nature, 225, 943 (1970).

Chihara, G. Pharmacia Review, 6, 119-131 (1981).

Coley, W.H. National Cancer Inst. Monograph, 44, 5 (1976).

Comfort, A. Aging - The Biology of Senescence. Edinburgh, Churchill Livingstone (1964).

Crowly, C. Curtis, H.J. Proc. Natl. Acad. Sci., 49, 626 (1963).

Currie G.A. and Bagshawe, K.D. Brit. Med. J., 1, 541 (1970).

Curtis, H.J. Science, 141, 686 (1963).

Cutler, R.G. Abst. 29th Ann. Meet. Gerontol. Soc. New York.(1976)

Cyong, J. Advances in Pharmacotherapy 2, 251 (1982).

Cyong, J.J. Gendai Toyo Igaku (Journal of Traditional Sino-Japanese Medicine) 5, 43 (1984).

Cyong, J. and Hanabusa, K. Phytochemistry 19, 2247 (1980).

Cyong, J. and Takahashi, M. Wakan Yaku Shinpojumu Kiroku (Proceedings of the Symposium on Oriental Medicines) 15, 150 (1981/82).

Deane H. W. and Fawcett, D.W. Anat. Rec. 113, 247 (1952).

De Backer, J.J. de Med. de Paris, 2, 276 (1897).

Diller, I.C., Mankowski, Z.T. and Fisher, M.E. Cancer Res., 23, 201 (1963).

Everson, T.C. and Cole, W.H. Spontaneous Regression of Cancer, W.B. Shunders (1966).

Field, A.K., Tytell, A.A., Lampson, G.P., Hilleman, M.R. Proc. Natl. Acad. Sci. U.S., 58, 1004 (1967).

Fujihira, K. J. of Japan Society for Oriental Medicine (Japan) 24, 465-479 (1973).

Fujihira, K. OHAI Bulletin 2, 1-22 (1977).

Foley, E.J. CancerRes., 13, 835 (1953).

Fujimura, J. and Osada, T. Japanese Journal of Primary Care 5, 285 (1982).

Gedick, P. and Fischer, R. Virchous Arch. Pathol. Anat. Physiol. 332, 431 (1959).

Gen, C.S. Chin J. Integr. Med. 6, 62-64 (1986).

Gitman, L., "Endocrines and Aging", Charles C. Thomas, Illinois (1967).

Gross, L. Cancer Res., 3, 326 (1943).

Halstead, B. W. and Hood, L.L. Eleutherococus senticosus (Siberian ginseng). Oriental Healing Arts Institute, Long Beach, 1984.

Hamperl, H. Virchows Arch. Pathol. Anat. Physiol. 292, 1 (1934).

Hamuro,J. and Hadding, U. Bitter-Suermann, Immunol., 34, 695 (1978).

Hamuro, J., Rollinghoff, M. and Wagner, H. Immunol., 39, 551 (1980).

Han, B.-H.,Han, Y.-N. and Park, M.-H. Chemical and Biochemical Studies on Antioxidant Components of Ginseng. In Advances in Chinese Medicinal Materials Research. Chang, H.M.,Yeung, H.W., Tso, W.W. and Koo, A. eds. World Scientific, Singapore. Philadelphia, 1985, p.485-498.

Hanabusa, K. et al. Planta Medica 29, 380 (1981).

Harman, D. J. Gerontol 11, 298 (1956).

Harman, D. Radiat. Res. 16, 753 (1962).

Hashimoto, H. Shibukawa, N., and Kojima, Y., Microbiol. Immunol. 22, 673 (1978).

Hiai, S. Effect of ginseng on endocrine system. In "Genseng", Oura, Kumagai, Shibata, Takagi, eds. Kyoritsu publish Co. Tokyo, 1981, pp 134-144.

Hikino, H. et al. Chemical and Pharmaceutical Bulletin 28, 2900 (1980).

Hirase, S., et al. Yakugaku Zasshi (Journal of the Pharmaceutical Society of Japan), 96, 419 (1976).

Hirose S. Fujin No Tomo, 83, 143-145 (1989).

Hooper, B. Clin. Exp. Immunol. 12,79 (1972).

Hou, Y., Ma, G., Wu, S., Li, Y. and Li, H. Chin. Med. J. 94, 35-40 (1981).

Hsu, H.-Y. et al, Oriental Materia Medica. Orienal Healing Arts Institute, Long Beach. 1986, p 640-641.

Issacs, A., Cox, R.A., Roten, Z. Lancet, ii, 113 (1963).

Issacs, A., Lindenmann, J. Proc. Roy. Soc. Biol., 147, 258 (1957)

Ishigami, J. Daisha (metabolism) 10, 590 (1973).

Ito, M. Nakashima, H., Baba, M., Pauwels, R., De Clercq, E., Shigeta, S. and Yamamoto, N. Antiviral Research, 7, 127-137 (1987).

Itokawa, H. et al. Tennen Yakubutsu no Kaihatsu to Oyo Shinpojumu Koenyoshishu (Abstracts of the Proceedings of the Symposium on the Development and Application of Natural Products) 3, 4 (1980).

Jin, Q. et al. Chin. J. Integr. Med. 5, 353-355 (1985).

Kamei, A., Hisada, T., and Iwata, S. J. Ocular Pharmacal. 3, 239-248 (1987).

Kaneko, M. Gendai Toyo Igaku (Journal of Traditional Sino-Japanese Medicine) 2, 28 (1981).

Kariyone, T. Saishin Shoyakugaku (Modern Pharmacognosy), 205-207. Tokyo, Hirokawa, 1964.

Kiangsu New Medical College, Chun yao ta tsu tien (Dictionary of Chinese Herbal Drugs), Science and Technology Press, Shanghai,1978

Kimura, M. Nihon Rinsho 25, 284 (1967).

Kimura, M. Proceeding of the 3rd International Ginseng Symposium pp 37 (1980). Korea Ginseng Research Institute, Seoul, Korea.

Kinoshita, J.H. Invest. Ophthalmol., 13, 713-724 (1974).

Kiyohara, H. et al. Wakan Iyaku Gakkai Koenyoshi (Absracts of the Annual Meeting of the Medical and Pharmaceutical Society for Wakan Yaku) 2, 60 (1985).

Kiyohara, H. et al. Nihon Seikagaku Gakkai Koenyoshi
    (Abstracts of of the Annual Meeting of the Japanese
    Biochemical Society) 58, 995 (1985).

Kohda, A. et al. Nihon Yakurigaku Zasshi (Journal of
    Japanese Pharmacology) 66, 366 (1970).

Kohda, A. et al. Nihon Yakurigaku Zasshi 67, 223 (1971).

Kohda, A. et al. Nihon Yakurigaku Zasshi 69, 889 (1973).

Kohda, A. and Nagai, H. Wakan Yaku Shinpojumu Kiroku 8,
    13 (1974/75).

Kokuda, T. et al. Tennen Yakubutsu no Kaihatsu to Oyo Shin-
    pojumu Koenyoshishu 2, 37 (1978).

Kohda, A. Chiryo-gaku (Biomedicine and Therapeutics) 7, 717
    (1981).

Kohda, A. et al. Nihon Yakurigaku Zasshi 78, 31 (1982).

Kohda, A. Pharma Medica 4, 93-100 (1986).

Kojima, Y. From the Discovery of Inteferon to Chinese
    Medicine. The 22nd Honomi Kanpo Seminar, Nagoya, 1984,
    p. 11-38.

Konno, C. et al. Planta Medica 35, 150 (1979).

Kosuga, T. et al. Yakugaku Zasshi (Journal of the
    Pharmaceutical Society of Japan) 98, 1370 (1978).

Kotani, T. e al. Nihon Yakugakkai Koenyoshishu (Abstracts of
    the Proceedings of the Pharmaceutical Society of Japan)
    103, 264 (1983).

Kubo Laboratory, Kinki University. Allergy to Kanpo (Allergy
    and Chinese Medicine) (Tokyo: Sanichi Shobo, 1984): 103-
    120.

Kubo, M. and Kotani, T. Kanpo I-Yakugaku (Chinese Herbal
    Medicine) (Tokyo: Hirokawa Publishing Co., 1984): 77, 88.

Kumagai, H. and Takada, Y. Wakan Yaku Shinpojumu Kiroku 8, 85 (1974).

Lewisohn, R., Leuchtenberger, C., Leuchtenberger, R., Laszuro, D. and Bloch, K. Cancer Res., 1, 799 (1941).

Lou, H. and Chen, C.H. J. Chin Internal Med. 3, 162-164 (1978).

Lu, Kuei-Sheng. Chung yo ko hsueh hua ta tzu tien (Dictionary of the Development of Chinese Medical Science). Hong Kong: 1954.

Maeda, Y.Y. and Chihara, G. Nature (London), 229, 634 (1971).

Maisin, J.R., Kondi-Tamba, A and Mattelin, G. Radiation Research, 105, 276 (1986).

Milas, L. and Mujagic, H.,Eur. J. Clin. Biol. Res., 17, 498 (1972).

Milch, R. Gerontologia 7, 129 (1963).

Mandrup-Poulsen, T. et al., Acta Pathol. Microbiol. Immunol. Scand. Sect. C 95, 55 (1987).

Makinodan, T. and Adler, W.H. Fed, Proc. 34, 153 (1975)

Meng, S.Y. Chin J. Integr. Med. 3, 374-375 (1983).

Meruels, D. Lavie, G. and Lavie, D. Proc. Natl. Acad. Sci. USA, 85, 5230-5234 (1988).

Miyake, N. Areruji (Allergy) 10, 131, (1961).

Miyazaki, T., et al. Carbohydrate Research, 65, 235 (1978).

Miyazaki, T., et al. Carbohydrate Research, 69, 165 (1979).

Miyazaki, T., et al. Chemical and Pharmaceutical Bulletin, 28, 3118 (1981a).

Miyazaki, T., et al. Chemical and Pharmaceutical Bulletin, 29, 316 (1981b).

Mizutami, K., Ohtani, K., Sumino, R., at al J. Pharmacobio-Dyn., 8, s-66 (1985).

Nagai,N. Yakugaku Zasshi 102, 109 (1982).

Nagai, T. et al. Nihon Shoyaku Gakkai Koenyoshi (Abstracts of the Annual Meeting of the Japanese Society of Pharmacognosy) 32, 6 (1985).

Nagoshi,N. and Nakano, K. Shoyakugaku Zasshi 30, 42-46 (1976).

Nakajima, S. et al. Wakan Yaku Shinpojumu Kiroku 13, 42 (1980).

Namba, T. Genshoku wakanyaku zukan (Colored Illustrations of Chinese Herbs). Hoikusha, Tokyo, 1980.

Nanking Pharmacy College. Zhong cao yao xue (Chinese Herbology) Jangsue: People's press, 1976.

Ninomiya, K. et al. Journal of Biochemistry 92, 413 (1982).

Nishii, K. et al. Wakan Yaku Shinpojumu Kiroku 15, 187 (1982).

Obata, H. et al. Virological Aspect (Japan) 1984.

Odashima, S., Nishikawa, K., Ohtsuka, A., Nakayabu, Y. and Abe, H. Europ. J. Cell Biol., 22, 396 (1980).

Ohtani, K., et al. Nihon Shoyaku Gakkai Koenyoshi, 32,4 (1985).

Okano, K. Kanpo no Rinsho (Practical Kanpo) 15, 11-12 nos. (1986).

Okuda, T., Yoshioka, Y., Ikekawa, T., Chihara,G. and Nishioka, K., Nature (London), New Biol., 208, 59 (1972).

Okuda, H. and Yoshida, R. Proceeding of the 3rd International Ginseng Symposium pp 53 (1980) Korea Ginseng Reseach Institute, Seoul, Korea.

Oura, H., Hirai, S., Odaka, Y. and Yokozawa, T. J. Biochem, 77, 1057 (1975).

Oura, H. and Yokozawa, T. Seikagaku 38, 689 (1966).

Pearson, J.W., Pearson, G.R., Gibson, W.T., Chermann, J.C. and Chirigos, M.A. Cancer Res., 32, 904 (1972).

Pelkov, W., Araneim, Forsch (Drug Res.) 11, 288 (1961).

Peng, Y. Bull. Chin. Materia Med. 8, 41-44 (1983).

Petkov, V. Arzneim-Forsch 28, 388 (1978).

Pruthi, J. R. Spices and Condiments: Chemistry, Microbiology, Technology: Chapter 2. New York: Academic Press, 1980.

Qian, Z., Li, Y. et al., Chin J. Integr Med 7, 268-269 (1987).

Quay, W.B., Gen. Comp. Endocrinol., 1, 211 (1963).

Reith, M.E.A., Schotman, P., Gipsen, W.H. & DeWied, D. Trends Biochem. Sci., 2, 56 (1975).

Roten, Z., Cox, R.A., Isaacs, A. Naure, 197, 564 (1963).

Ruprecht, R.M. O'Brien, L.G., Rossini, L.D. & Nusinoff-Lehrman, S. Nature (London) 323, 467-469 (1986).

Sacher, G.A., Relation of lifespan to brain weight and body wight in mammals. In wolstenholme, G.E.W. and O'Connor, M. (ed.) Ciba Foundation Coll. on Aging Vol. 5, p.115, London, Churchill.(1959)

Saito, Y. Shoyaku Bunseki Toronkai Koenyoshishu (Abstracts of the Forum for the Discussion of Pharmacognostic Analysis) 42(1982).

Saito, H. Int. Symp. Gerontology (Lugano) p.65 (1976).

Saito, H. and Bao, T. OHAI Bull. 11, 481 (1986).

Sasaki, T. et al. Carbohydrate Research 47, 99 (1976).

Sato, S. The effect of ginseng saponins on experimental ulceration. In "Genseng", Oura, Kumagai, Shibata, Takagi, ed. Kyoritsu publish C., Tokyo, 1981, pp 157.

Sato, S., Kojima, A. Karasawa, H. et al. Oyo Yakuri (Applied Pharmacology) 20, 425 (1980).

Sekiguchi, S. et al. Gendai Igaku (Jap), 14, 341 (1982).

Shen Nung Pen tsao ching ("Shen Nung's Herbal"). Han dynasty, 25 B.C.-220 A.D. [Modern edition by Sun, Hsin-yen and Sun, Hsin-i (Hong Kong: Commercial Press, 1955, and Taipei: Chunghua Book Co., 1965)].

Shibata, M., J. Traditional Sino-Japanese Med. 1, 37-40 (1980). (in Japanese).

Shibata, S. et al. Arerugi (Allergy) 8, 254 (1959).

Shibata S., in Wangner H., Wolff P., ed. New Natural Products and Plant Drugs with Pharmacological, Biological or Therapeutical Activity. Berlin Heidelberg: Springer-Verlag, 1977; pp177-196.

Smith, M.O. World Congress of Acupuncture and Natural Medicine, Beijing, Novemberr, 1987.

Smith, R.J. Am Col. Trad. Chin. Med. 1(2), 20-29 (1985).

Sokai Editorial Department. Roka O fusegu Kanpo no meiyaku (Popular Kanpo for the Prevention of Aging): 188. Tokyo: Makino, 1979.

Stlehler, B.L., "Time, Cells and Aging", Acad. Press, N.Y.(1962)

Stubel, H. Arch. Gesamte Physiol. 142, 1 (1911).

Sulkin, N.M. Assoc. Gerontol. 3rd Cong. P. 156 (1955).

Takagi, K. et al. Wakan yakubutsugaku (The Pharmacology of Chinese Medicinal Herbs), Nanzando, Tokyo, 1982.

Takahashi, M. Planta Medica, 51, 100 (1985).

Tamamura, S., Shibukawa, N., Kojima, Y. J. Med. Pharm. Wakan-Yaku 1, 72-73 (1984).

Tanno, Y. Nihon Yakubutsugaku Zasshi (Journal of Japanese Pharmaceuticals) 33, 263 (1941).

Tao, J. et al. Zongchenyao Yangjue (Studies in Chinese Herbal Medicine) 6, 5 (1981).

Tomimori, T. and Yoshimoto, M. Shoyakugaku Zasshi, 34, 138-144 (1980).

Tashiro, S. Kanpo Igaku (Kanpo Medicine) 9, 16 (1985).

Tsung, P.-K. OHAI Bull. 12, 1-10 (1987).

Tsung, P.-K, and Hsu, H.-Y. Immunology and Chinese Herbal Medicine. Oriental Healing Arts Institute, Long Beach, 1986.

Ueno, Y. et al. Carbohydrate Research 101, 160 (1982).

Ukai, S. et al. Carbohydrate Research 105, 237 (1982).

U.S., Patent 4675318, 1987.

Usuki, S. Am. J. Chinese Med. 14, 37-45 (1986).

Varma, S.D. and Kinoshita, J.H. Biochim. Biophys. Acta., 338, 632-640, (1974).

Walford, R. L. The Immunologic Theory of Aging: Current status. Fed. Proc. Am. Soc. Exp. Biol. 33, 2020 (1974).

Walford, R. L. The Immunologic theory of Aging. Williams & Willkins, Baltimore (1969).

Wang, Ping. Huang ti nei ching (The Yellow Emperor's Treatise on Internal Medicine). Tang dynasty(762 A.D.). [English Translations by Veith, Ilza (Su wen secttion only, Berkeley: Univ. of California Press, 1949) and Lu, Henry C. (Vancouver, B.C.:Academy of Oriental Heritage, 1978).]

Yagi, A. et al. Wakan Yaku Shinpojumu Kiroku 13, 72 (1980).

Yagi, A. et al. Yakugaku Zasshi 101, 700 (1981).

Yamada, H. et al. Carbohydrate Research 125, 107 (1984).

Yamada, H. et al. International Journal of Immunopharmacology 7, 358 (1985).

Yamada, H. et al. Molecular Immunology 22, 295 (1985).

Yamada, H. et al. Planta Medica 51, 121 (1985).

Yamada, H. et al. Nihon Yakugaku Gakkai Koenyoshi (Abstracts of the Annual Meeting of the Japanese Pharmaceutical Society) 105, 446 (1985).

Yamada, H. et. al. International Journal of Immunopharmacology [in press].

Yamada, H., Cyong, J.-C. et al., Planta Medica 48, 117-204 (1984).

Yamada, H. Cyong, J. and Ohtsuka, Y. OHAI Bull. 12, 11-23 (1987).

Yamahara, J. et al. Yakugaku Zasshi 102, 881 (1982).

Yamamoto, M., Kumagai A., Yamamura Y. Arzneim-Forsch 25, 1021-1023 (1975).

Yamamoto, M., Kumagai A., Yamamura Y. Arzneim-Forsch 25, 1240-1243 (1975).

Yamamoto, M., Kumagai, A. and Yamamura, Y. Arznein-Forsch., 27, 1404(1977).

Yamamoto, M., Masaka, M., Yamada, K., Hayashi, Y., Hirai, A., and Kumagai, A. Arzneimittelforschung, 27, 1169 (1977).

Yamamoto, M., Uemura, T., Nakama, S. et al. J. Med. Pharm. Soc. for WAKAN-YAKU 2, 377 (1985).

Yamauchi, K. and Tsunematsu, T. Wakan 'Yaku Shinpojumu Kiroku (Proceedings of the Wakan 'Yaku Symposium) 15, 29 (1981/82).

Yan, Shuchang. Chin J. Integr. Med. 8, 141-143 (1988).

Yata, N. and Tanaka, O. OHAI Bull. 13, 13-22 (1988).

Yonezawa, M. Radiation Damage and Ginseng. In "Ginseng '85, the basic and clinic studies". Kumagai, A., Oura, H., and Okuda, H. eds. Kyoritsu Publishing Co., Tokyo, 1985, p.71-83.

Yonezawa, M., Hosokawa Y., Katoh, N., and Takeda A. OHAI Bull., 12, 39-49 (1987).

Yonezawa, M. Katoh, N. and Takeda, A. Shoyakugaku Zasshi, 39, 139 (1981a).

Yonezawa, M. Katoh, N. and Takeda, A. J. Radiat. Res., 22, 336 (1981b).

Index

M

Appendix 1

Chinese Herbal Names

Name	Pin-yin	Chinese Name
Abrus	Ji-Gu-Cao	鷄骨草
Abutilon	Dong-Kui-Zi	冬葵子
Acanthopanax	Wu-Jia-Pi	五加皮
Achyranthes	Niu-Xi	牛膝
Aconite(processed)	Fu-Zi	附子(加工)
Aconite(roasted)	Fu-Zi	附子(炮)
Acorus	Chang-Pu	菖蒲
Acronychia	Jiang-Zhen-Xiang	降真香
Aeginetia	Guan-Zheng-Huang	官真癀
Agastache	Huo-Xiang	藿香
Agrimony	Xian-He-Cao	仙鶴草
Ailanthus Root	Bai-Chun-Pi	白椿皮
Akebia	Mu-Tong	木通
Albizzia	He-Huan-Pi	合歡皮
Alisma	Ze-Xie	澤瀉
Allium	Cong-Bai	葱白
Alpinia Fruits	Yi-Zhi-Ren	益智仁
Ampelopsis	Bai-Lian	白薇
Anemarrhena	Zhi-Mu	知母
Anemone	Bai-Tou-Weng	白頭翁
Angelica	Bai-Zhi	白芷

Name	Pin-yin	Chinese Name
Anteater Scales	Chuan-Shan-Jia	穿山甲
Apricot Seed	Xing-Ren	杏仁
Aquilaria	Chen-Xiang	沈香
Arctium	Niu-Bang-Zi	牛蒡子
Ardisia	Zou-Mai-Tai	走馬胎
Areca Peel	Da-Fu-Pi	大腹皮
Areca Seed	Bing-Lang-Zi	檳榔子
Arisaema	Tian-Nan-Xing	天南星
Aristolochia	Ma-Dou-Ling	馬兜鈴
Artemisia	Ai-Ye	艾葉
Artemisia Root	Ai-Tou	艾頭
Asarum	Xi-Xin	細辛
Asparagus	Tian-Men-Dong	天門冬
Aster	Zi-Wan	紫菀
Astragalus	Huang-Qi	黃芪
Astragalus Seed	Sha-Yuan-Zi	沙苑子
Atractylodes	Cang-Zhu	蒼术
Atractylodes(white)	Bai-Zhu	白术
Bakeri	Xie-Bai	薤白
Bamboo(Shavings)	Zhu-Ru	竹茹
Baphicacanthis [Isatis]	Da-Qing-Ye	大青葉
Belamcanda	She-Gan	射干
Benincasa	Dong-Gua-Zi	冬瓜子
Biota	Bo-Zi-Ren	柏子仁
Biota Tops	Ce-Bo-Ye	側柏葉

Name	Pin-yin	Chinese Name
Birthwort	Tian-Xian-Teng	天仙藤
Blechnum	Guan-Zhong	貫衆
Bletilla	Bai-Ji	白芨
Blue Citrus	Qing-Pi	青皮
Blumea	Da-Feng-Cao	大風草
Brassica[Sinapsis]	Bai-Jie-Zi	白芥子
Broussonetia	Chu-Shi-Zi	楮實子
Brucea	Ku-Shen-Zi	苦參子
Buddleia	Mi-Meng-Hua	密蒙花
Bulrush	Pu-Huang	蒲黄
Bupleurum	Chai-Hu	柴胡
Calamus Gum	Xue-Jie	血竭
Campsis	Ling-Xiao-Hua	凌霄花
Capillaris	Yin-Chen-Hao	茵陳蒿
Cardamon	Suo-Sha	縮砂
Carthamus	Hong-Hua	紅花
Cassia Seed	Jue-Ming-Zi	決明子
Celastrus	Chuan-Shan-Long	穿山龍
Celosia	Qing-Xiang-Zi	青箱子
Centipeda	E-Bu-Shi-Cao	鵝不食草
Centranthera	Jin-Suo-Chi	金鎖匙
Chaenomeles	Mu-Gua	木瓜
Changium	Ming-Dang-Shen	明黨參
Chiang-Huo	Qiang-Huo	羌活
Chih-Ko	Zhi-Ko	枳殼

Name	Pin-yin	Chinese Name
Chih-Shih	Zhi-Shi	枳實
Chin-Chiu	Qin-Jiao	秦艽
Ching-Hao	Qing-Hao	青蒿
Chrysanthemum	Ju-Hua	菊花
Cibotium	Gou-Ji	狗脊
Cicada	Chan-Tui	蟬蛻
Cimicifuga	Sheng-Ma	升麻
Cinnamon Bark	Gui-Pi	桂皮
Cinnamon Twigs	Gui-Zhi	桂枝
Cirsium	Da-Xiao-Ji	大小薊
Cistanche	Rou-Cong-Rong	肉蓯蓉
Citrus	Chen-Pi	陳皮
Citrus Seed	Ju-He	橘核
Clematis	Wei-Ling-Xian	威靈仙
Clove	Ding-Xiang	丁香
Cluster	Bai-Dou-Kou	白豆蔻
Cnidium	Chuan-Xiong	川芎
Cnidium Fruit	She-Chuang-Zi	蛇床子
Cocculus	Niu-Ru-Shi	牛入石
Cockscomb	Ji-Guan-Hua	鷄冠花
Codonopsis	Dang-Shen	黨參
Coix	Yi-Yi-Ren	薏苡仁
Coptis	Huang-Lian	黄連
Corn Stigma	Yu-Mi-Xu	玉米須
Cornus	Shan-Zhu-Yu	山茱萸

Name	Pin-yin	Chinese Name
Corydalis	Yan-Hu-Suo	延胡索
Crataegus	Shan-Zha	山楂
Cudrania	Da-Ding-Huang	大丁癀
Curculigo	Xian-Mao	仙茅
Curcuma	Jiang-Huang	姜黄
Cuscuta	Tu-Si-Zi	菟絲子
Cuttlebone	Hai-Piao-Xiao	海螵蛸
Cyclina	Hai-Ge-Fen	海蛤粉
Cynanchum	Bai-Qian	白前
Cynomorium	Suo-Yang	鎖陽
Cyperus	Xiang-Fu-Zi	香附子
Dandelion	Pu-Gong-Ying	蒲公英
Datura	Yang-Jin-Hua	洋金花
Dendrobium	Shi-Hu	石斛
Desmodium	Jin-Qian-Cao	金錢草
Dianthus	Qu-Mai	瞿麥
Dichondra	Ma-Ti-Jin	馬蹄金
Dichroa Root	Chang-Shan	常山
Digenea	Hai-Ren-Cao	海人草
Dioscorea	Shan-Yao	山藥
Dipsacus	Xu-Duan	續斷
Dolichos	Bai-Pian-Dou	白扁豆
Dolichos Root	Rou-Dou-Gen	肉豆根
Dragon Bone	Long-Gu	龍骨
Drynaria	Gu-Sui-Bu	骨碎補

Name	Pin-yin	Chinese Name
Earthworm	Di-Long	地龍
Echinops	Lou-Lu	漏蘆
Eclipta	Han-Lian-Cao	旱蓮草
Elaeagnus	Yi-Wu-Gen	梔梧根
Elephantopi	Di-Dan-Tou	地膽頭
Elsholtzia	Xiang-Ru	香薷
Epimedium	Yin-Yang-Huo	淫羊藿
Equisetum	Mu-Zei	木賊
Eriobotrya	Pi-Pa-Ye	枇杷葉
Eriocaulon	Gu-Jing	穀精
Eucommia	Du-Zhong	杜仲
Eupatorium	Pei-Lan	佩蘭
Euryale	Qian-Shi	芡實
Evodia	Wu-Zhu-Yu	吳茱萸
Fagopyrum	Qiao-Mai	蕎麥
Fennel	Xiao-Hui-Xiang	小茴香
Ficus	Feng-Bu-Dong	風不動
Finger crtron	Fo-Shou-Gan	佛手柑
Forsythia	Lian-Qiao	連翹
Fraxinella	Bai-Xian-Pi	白鮮皮
Fraxinus	Qin-Pi	秦皮
Fritillaria	Bei-Mu	貝母
Fu-Shen	Fu-Shen	茯神
Futokadsura	Da-Feng-Teng	大風藤
Galanga	Liang-Jiang	良姜

Name	Pin-yin	Chinese Name
Gall	Wu-Bei-Zi	五倍子
Gambir [Uncaria]	Diao-Teng-Gou	釣藤鈎
Gardenia	Zhi-Zi	梔子
Garlic	Da-Suan	大蒜
Gastrodia	Tian-Ma	天麻
Gelatin	A-Jiao	阿膠
Gentiana	Long-Dan	龍膽
Germinated Rice	Gu-Ya	穀芽
Ginger(dried)	Gan-Jiang	乾姜
Ginger(fresh)	Sheng-Jiang	生姜
Ginkgo	Yin-Xing	銀杏
Ginseng	Ren-Shen	人參
Gleditsia	Zao-Jia	皂角
Gleditsia Spine	Zao-Ci	皂刺
Glehnia	Bei-Sha-Shen	北沙參
Granatum Rind	Shi-Liu-Pi	石榴皮
Gymnema	Wu-Xue-Teng	武靴藤
Gypsum	Shi-Gao	石膏
Haematite	Dai-Zhe-Shi	代赭石
Haliotis	Shi-Jue-Ming	石決明
Helminthostachys	Di-Wu-Song	地蜈蚣
Ho-Shou-Wu	He-Shou-Wu	何首烏
Hoelen	Fu-Ling	茯苓
Hoelen(red)	Chi-Ling	赤苓
Homalomena	Qian-Nian-Jian	千年健

Name	Pin-yin	Chinese Name
Houttuynia	Yu-Xing-Cao	魚腥草
Hovenia	Zhi-Ju-Zi	枳俱子
Ilex	Wan-Dian-Jin	萬點金
Imperata	Bai-Mao-Gen	白茅根
Inula	Xuan-Fu-Hua	旋覆花
Isatis Root	Ban-Lan-Gen	板藍根
Jujube	Da-Zao	大棗
Juncus	Deng-Xin-Cao	燈心草
Kadsura	Hong-Gu-She	紅骨蛇
Kaempferia	Shan-Nai	山奈
Kaki	Shi-Di	柿蒂
Kao-Pen	Gao-Ben	蒿本
Kaolin	Chi-Shi-Zhi	赤石脂
Kochia	Di-Fu-Zi	地膚子
Laminaria	Hai-Dai	海帶
Lashio Sphaera	Ma-Bo	馬勃
Leech	Shui-Zhi	水蛭
Leek	Jiu-Zi	韭子
Leonurus	Yi-Mu-Cao	益母草
Leonurus Seed	Chong-Wei-Zi	茺蔚子
Lepidium	Ting-Li-Zi	葶藶子
Leucadis	Bai-Hua-Zi-Cao	白花仔草
Licorice	Gan-Cao	甘草
Ligustrum	Nu-Zhen-Zi	女貞子
Lily	Bai-He	百合

Name	Pin-yin	Chinese Name
Limonite	Yu-Yu-Liang	禹餘糧
Lindera	Wu-Yao	烏藥
Lindernia	Ding-Jing-Cao	定經草
Linum	Ma-Zi-Ren	麻子仁
Lippia	Ya-She-Huang	鴨舌癀
Liquidambar	Lu-Lu-Tong	路路通
Litchi Seed	Li-Zhi-He	荔枝核
Lithospermum	Zi-Cao	紫草
Longan Flower	Long-Yan-Hua	龍眼花
Lonicera	Jin-Yin-Hua	金銀花
Lonicera Stem	Ren-Dong-Teng	忍冬藤
Lophatherum	Dan-Zhu-Ye	淡竹葉
Loranthus	Sang-Ji-Sheng	桑寄生
Lotus Embryo	Lian-Zi-Xin	蓮子心
Lotus Fruits	Shi-Lian-Zi	石蓮子
Lotus Leaf	Lian-Ye	蓮葉
Lotus Node	Ou-Jie	藕節
Lotus Receptacles	Lian-Fang	蓮房
Lotus Seed	Lian-Zi	蓮子
Lotus Stamen	Lian-Xu	蓮須
Ludwigia	Shui-Deng-Xiang	水燈香
Luffa Fiber	Si-Gua-Luo	絲瓜絡
Lycium Bark	Di-Gu-Pi	地骨皮
Lycium Fruit	Gou-Qi-Zi	枸杞子
Lycium Root	Gou-Qi-Gen	枸杞根

Name	Pin-yin	Chinese Name
Lycopodium	Jin-Bu-Huan	金不換
Lycopus	Ze-Lan	澤蘭
Lygodium	Hai-Jin-Sha	海金砂
Ma-Huang	Ma-Huang	麻黃
Ma-Huang Root	Ma-Huang Gen	麻黃根
Madder	Qian-Cao-Gen	茜草根
Magnolia Bark	Hou-Pu	厚朴
Magnolia Flower	Xin-Yi	辛夷
Malt	Mai-Ya	麥芽
Manganite	Wu-Ming-I	無名異
Mantis	Sang-Piao-Xiao	桑螵蛸
Mastic	Ru-Xiang	乳香
Melia	Chuan-Lian-Zi	川楝子
Mentha	Bo-He	薄荷
Millettia	Ji-Xue-Deng	鷄血藤
Mirabilitum	Mang-Xiao	芒硝
Moghania	Yi-Tiao-Gen	一條根
Morinda	Ba-Ji-Tian	巴戟天
Morus Bark	Sang-Bai-Pi	桑白皮
Morus Branch	Sang-Chi	桑枝
Morus Leaves	Sang-Ye	桑葉
Moutan	Mu-Dan-Pi	牡丹皮
Mugwort	Liu-Ji-Nu	劉寄奴
Mume	Wu-Mei	烏梅
Myristicae	Rou-Dou-Kou	肉豆蔻

Name	Pin-yin	Chinese Name
Myrrh	Mo-Yao	沒藥
Nei-Chin	Nei-Jin	鷄內金
Ocimum	Jiu-Ceng-Ta	九層塔
Oldenlandia	Bai-Hua-She-She-Cao	白花蛇舌草
Omphalia	Lei-Wan	雷丸
Ophiopogon	Mai-Men-Dong	麥門冬
Orange Peel	Ju-Hong	橘紅
Oroxylum	Gu-Zhi-Hua	故紙花
Orthosiphon	Hua-Shi-Cao	化石草
Oryza	Jing-Mi	粳米
Oyster Shell	Mu-Li	牡蠣
Paederia	Ji-Xiang-Teng	鷄香藤
Pai-Wei	Bai-Wei	白薇
Peony	Shao-Yao	芍藥
Peony Red	Chi-Shao	赤芍
Perilla Leaves	Zi-Su-Ye	紫蘇葉
Perilla Seed	Zi-Su-Zi	紫蘇子
Perilla Stalk	Su-Geng	蘇梗
Persica	Tao-Ren	桃仁
Peucedanum	Qian-Hu	前胡
Pharbitis	Qian-Niu-Zi	牽牛子
Phaseolus	Chi-Xiao-Dou	赤小豆
Phellodendron	Huang-Bo	黃柏
Phragmites	Lu-Gen	蘆根
Picrorrhizae Rhizoma	Hu-Huang-Lian	胡黃連

Name	Pin-yin	Chinese Name
Pig Gallbladder	Zhu-Tan	猪膽
Pileostegia	Bai-Chun-Gen	白椿根
Pine Nodes	Song-Jie	松節
Pinellia	Ban-Xia	半夏
Piper	Pi-Bo	蓽撥
Pittosporum	Qi-Li-Xiang	七里香
Placenta	Zi-He-Che	紫河車
Plantago	Che-Qian-Zi	車前子
Plantain	Che-Chian-Cao	車前草
Platycodon	Jie-Geng	桔梗
Plum Seed	Yu-Li-Ren	郁李仁
Pogonatherum	Bi-Zi-Cao	筆仔草
Polygala	Yuan-Zhi	遠志
Polygonatum	Yu-Zhu	玉竹
Polygonatum Roots	Huang-Jing	黄精
Polygonum	Bian-Xu	扁蓄
Polygonum Stem	Ye-Jiao-Teng	夜交藤
Polyporus	Zhu-Ling	猪苓
Polygala Herba	Tie-Diao-Gan	鐵釣竿
Prickly Ash	Niao-Bu-Su	鳥不宿
Prinsepia	Rui-Ren	蕤仁
Prunella	Xia-Ku-Cao	夏枯草
Psoralea	Bu-Gu-Zhi	補骨脂
Pteris	Feng-Wei-Cao	鳳尾草
Pteropous	Wu-Ling-Zhi	五靈脂

Name	Pin-yin	Chinese Name
Pueraria	Ge-Gen	葛根
Pumice	Hai-Fu-Shi	海浮石
Pyrite	Zi-Ran-Tong	自然銅
Quisqualis	Shi-Jun-Zi	使君子
Raphanus	Lai-Fu-Zi	萊服子
Rauwolfia	Bai-Hua-Lian	白花蓮
Rehmannia	Sheng-Di-Huang	生地黃
Rehmannia Cooked	Shu-Di-Huang	熟地黃
Rhubarb	Da-Huang	大黃
Rosa(cherokee)	Jing-Ying-Zi	金櫻子
Rose	Xiao-Jin-Ying	小金櫻
Rostellularia	Shu-Wai-Huang	鼠尾癀
Rubus	Fu-Pen-Zi	覆盆子
Salvia	Dan-Shen	丹參
Sanguisorba	Di-Yu	地榆
Santalum	Tan-Xiang	檀香
Sappan Wood	Su-Mu	蘇木
Sargassum	Hai-Zao	海藻
Saussurea	Mu-Xiang	木香
Schizandra	Wu-We-Zi	五味子
Schizonepeta	Jing-Jie	荊芥
Scirpus [Sparganium]	San-Ling	三稜
Scorpion	Quan-Xie	全殭
Scrophularia	Xuan-Shen	玄參
Scute	Huang-Qin	黃芩

Name	Pin-yin	Chinese Name
Scute Herba	Ban-Zhi-Lian	半枝蓮
Securinegae	Hong-Ci-Cong	紅刺蔥
Selaginella	Long-Lin-Cao	龍鱗草
Senecio	Qian-Li-Guang	千里光
Senna	Fan-Xie-Ye	番瀉葉
Sesame	Hu-Ma-Ren	胡麻仁
Shen-Chu	Shen-Qu	神麴
Siegesbeckia	Xi-Qian-Cao	豨簽草
Siler	Fang-Feng	防風
Silkworm	Bai-Jiang-Can	白殭蠶
Smilax	Tu-Fu-Ling	土茯苓
Soja	Dan-Dou-Chi	淡豆豉
Solanum	Huang-Shui-Qie	黃水茄
Sophora	Huai-Hua	槐花
Sophora Root	Ku-Shen	苦參
Stemona	Bai-bu	百部
Stephania	Fang-Chi	防己
Sterculia	Pang-Da-Hai	胖大海
Subprostrata	Shan-Dou-Gen	山豆根
Talc	Hua-Shi	滑石
Tang-Kuei	Dang-Gui	當歸
Terminalia	Ke-Zi	訶子
Tetrapanax	Tong-Cao	通草
Thlaspi	Bai-Jiang-Cao	敗醬草
Thymifolia	Zhu-Zi-Cao	珠仔草

Name	Pin-yin	Chinese Name
Tokoro	Bi-Jie	萆薢
Torreya	Fei-Zi	榧子
Tortoise Shell	Gui-Pan	龜板
Tou-Ku-Tsao	Tou-Su-Cao	透骨草
Tribulus	Ji-Li	蒺藜
Trichosanthes Fruit	Gua-Lou	栝樓
Trichosanthes Peel	Gua-Lou-Pi	栝樓皮
Trichosanthes Root	Gua-Lou-Gen	栝樓根
Trichosanthes Seed	Gua-Lou-Ren	栝樓仁
Tsao-Ko	Cao-Guo	草果
Tsao-Tou-Kou	Cao-Dou-Kou	草豆蔻
Tu-Huo	Du-Huo	獨活
Tumeric	Yu-Jin	郁金
Turtle Shell	Bie-Jia	鱉甲
Tussilago	Kuan-Dong-Hua	款冬花
Uiva	Kun-Bu	昆布
Vaccaria	Wang-Bu-Liu-Xing	王不留行
Vanieria	Huang-Jin-Gui	黃金桂
Verbena	Ma-Bian-Cao	馬鞭草
Veronica	Yi-Zhi-Xiang	一枝香
Viola	Zi-Hua-Di-Ding	紫花地丁
Vitex	Man-Jing-Zi	蔓荊子
Vitex Root	Pu-Jiang-Gen	埔姜根
Walnut	Hu-Tao-Rou	胡桃仁
Wheat	Fu-Xiao-Mai	浮小麥

Name	Pin-yin	Chinese Name
Xanthium	Cang-Er-Zi	蒼耳子
Zanthoxylum	Shan-Jiao	山椒
Zedoaria	E-Shu	莪术
Zizyphus	Suan-Zao-Ren	酸棗仁

Appendix 2

Chinese Herbal Formulas
By English Names, Chinese Pinyin, And Japanese Names.

English name	Pinyin	Japanese name
Achyanthes & plantago formula	niuche shenqi wan	gusya-zinki-gan
Aconite & oryza combination	fuzi gengmi tang	fusi-kobei-to
Aaconite combination	fuzi tang	fusi-to
Aconite, ginger & licorice combination	sini tang	sigyaku-to
Aconite, ginseng & ginger combination	fuzi lizhong tang	fusi-richu-to
Adenophora & ophiopogon combination	shashen maidong tang	sasan-bakuto-to
Agastache formula	huoxiang zhengqi san	kakko-shoki-sa
Alisma combination	zexie tang	takusha-to
Anemarrhena, phellodendron & rehmannia formula	zhi bo bawei wan	chiheki-hachimi-gan

Anemone combination	baitouweng tang	hakuto-oh-to
Angelica & mastic combination	xianfan huoming yin	senhou-katsume-in
Apricot seed & linum formula	maziren wan	masi-nin-gan
Apricot seed & perilla formula	xing su san	kyoso-san
Aquilaria & gastrodia combination	chenxiang tianma tang	chinko-tenma-to
Aquilaria & perilla formula	sanhe san	sanwa san
Arctium combination	qingyan lige tang	seiin-rikaku-to
Areca & evodia combination	bianzhi xingi yin	hensei-sinki-in
Areca seed & chaenomeless formula	jiming san	keimei-san
Areca seed combination	jiu bing wu fu tang	kyuhin-gofuku-to
Asarum & cimicifuga formula	lixiao san	rikko-san
Aster combinaiton	ziwan tang	shien-to

Astragalus & aconite formula	shiwei cuo san	jyumiza-san
Astragalus & atractylodes combination	qingshu yiqi tang	seisyo-ekki-to
Astragalus & cinnamon 5 herb combination	huangqi guizhi wuwu tang	ogi-keishi-gomotsu-to
Astragalus & Platycodon formula	qianjin neituo san	senkin-naitaku-san
Astragalus & t.s. formula	huangqi biejia san	ogi-kikko-san
Astragalus & zizyphus formula	yang xin tang	yosin-to
Astragalus combination	huangqi jianzhong tang	ogi-kenchu-to
Atractylodes & arisaema combination	ershu tang	nizyutu-to
Atractylodes & cardamon combination	chuansi junzi tang	zensi-kunsi-to
Atractylodes & pueraria formula	qianshi baishu san	sensi-hakuzyutu- to
Atractylodes & setaria combination	wei feng tang	ifu-to

Atractylodes combination	yuebi jiashu tang	eppi-ka-zyutu-to
Aurantium & bamboo combination	jupi zhuru tang	kippi-tikunyo-to
Bamboo & ginseng combination	zhuru wendan tang	tikuzyo-untan-to
Bamboo leaves & gypsum combination	zhuye shiqao tang	tikuyo-sekko-to
Biota & achyranthes formula	boziren wan	hakusi-jin-gan
Blue dragon combination (minor)	xiao qinglong tang	syo-seiryu-to
Bupleurum & chih-shih formula	sini san	sigyaku-san
Bupleurum & cinnamon combination	chaihu guizhi tang	saiko-keisi-to
Bupleurum & cyperus combination	chaihu shugan tang	saiko-sokan-to
Bupleurum & d.b. combination	chaihu jia longgu muli tang	saiko-ka-ryukotu-borei-to
Bupleurum & evodia combination	shugan tang	sokan-to
Bupleurum & hoelen combination	chai ling tang	sairei-to

Bupleurum & paeonia formula	jiawei xiaoyao san	kami-syoyo-san
Bupleurum & pueraria combination	chai ge jieji tang	saikatsu-kaiki-to
Bupleurum & rehmannia combination	chaihu qinggan tang	saiko-seikan-to
Bupleurum & schizonepeta formula	shiwei baidu tang	zyumi-haidoku-to
Bupleurum & scute combination	chaixian tang	saikan-to
Bupleurum formula	yigan san	yoku-kan-san
Bupleurum, cinnamon & ginger combination	chaihu guizhi ganjiang tang	saiko-keisi-kankyo-to
Bupleurum, citrus & pinellia formula	yigan san jia chenpi banxia	yoku-kan-san-ka-tinpi-hange
Bupleurum, paeonia & six major herbs combination	chai shao liujunzi tang	saisyaku-rikkunsi-to
Capillaris & hoelen five formula	yinchen wuling san	intin-gorei-san
Capillaris combination	yinchenhao tang	intin-ko-to
Cardamon & fennel formula	anzhong san	antyu-san

Cardamon combiantion	liuhe tang	rokuwa-to
Chianghuo & turmeric combinaiton	juanbi tang	shoku-hi-to
Chianghuo combination	jiuwei jianghuo tang	kumi-kyokatu-to
Chih-shih & cardamon combinaiton	zhi suo erchen tang	kishuku-nichin-to
Chih-shih & peony formula	zhishi shaoyao san	kijitu-syakuyaku-san
Chih-shih & t.s. formula	qinjiao biejia san	sinkyu-kikko-san
Chih-shih, bakeri & cinnamon combiantion	zhishi xiebai guizhi tang	kijitsu-senhaku-keisi-to
Chrysanthemum combination	zishen mingmu tang	jijin-meimoku-to
Cimicifuga & pueraria combination	shengma gegen tang	syoma-kakkon-to
Cimicifuga combination	yizi tang	otuzi-to
Cinnamon & aconite combination	guizhi jia fuzi tang	keisi-ka-fusi-to

Cinnamon & anemarrhena combiantion	guizhi shaoyao zhimu tang	keisi-syakuyaku-chimo-to
Cinnamon & angelica formula	shangzhongxia tong- yong tongfeng wan	jochuge-tsuyo-tsufu-gan
Cinnamon & astragalus combination	guizhi jia huangqi tang	keisi-ka-ogi-to
Cinnamon & atractylodes combination	guizhi jia ling shu fu tang	keisi-ka-reizyutubu-to
Cinnamon & d.b. combination	guizhi jia longgu muli tang	keisi-ka-ryukotu-borei-to
Cinnamon & d.d.o. combinaiton	guizhi qu shaoyao jia shuqi longgu muli tang	keisi-kyo-syakuyaku-ka-shokushitu-ryukotu-borei-to
Cinnamon & ginseng combination	guizhi renshen tang	keisi-ninzin-to
Cinnamon & hoelen formula	guizhi fuling wan	keisi-bukuryo-gan
Cinnamon & ma-huang combination	guizhi mahuang geban tang	keisi-mao-kakuhan-to
Cinnamon & poeny combination	guizhi jia shaoyao tang	keisi-ka-syakuyaku-to

Cinnamon & pueraria combination	guizhi jia gegen tang	keisi-ka-kakkon-to
Cinnamon combination	guizhi tang	keisi-to
Cinnamon five herbs combination	guizhi wuwu tang	keisi-gomotsu-to
Cinnamon, atractylodes & aconite combinaiton	guizhi jia shu fu tang	keisi-ka-zyutubu-to
Cinnamon, magnolia & apricot seed combination	guizhi jia houpu xingren tang	keisi-ka-koboku-kyonin-to
Cinnamon, poeny & rhubarb combination	guizhi jia shaoyao dahuang tang	keisi-ka-syakuyaku-daio-to
Citrus & crataegus formula	bao he wan	howa-gan
Citrus & perilla combination	fengxinqi yin	bunsinki-in
Citrus & pinellia combination	er chen tang	nitin-to
Clematis & charthamus formula	shujin lian san	jokin-ritsuan-san
Clematis & stephania	shujing huoxie tang	sokei-kakketu-to

Clove & hoelen combination	dingxiang fuling tang	choka-bukuryo-to
Cnidium & moutan combination	qingre huxie tang	seinetsu-hoki-to
Cnidium & rehmannia combination	xiong gui diaoxie	kyuki-choketsu-in
Cnidium & tea formula	chuanxiong chadiao san	senkyu-tyatyo-san
Coix combination	yiyiren tang	yokuinin-to
Coix, aconite, thlaspi formula	yiyiren fuzi baijiang san	yokuijin-fusi-haisho-san
Coptis & gelatin combination	huanglian ajiao tang	oren-akyo-to
Coptis & rehmannia formula	quingwei san	sei-i-san
Coptis & rhubarb combination	sanhuang xiexin tang	sano-syasin-to
Coptis & scute combination	huanglian jiedu tang	oren-gedoku-to
Coptis combinaiton	huanglian tang	oren-to
Coptis, hoelen & atractylodes combination	weichang san	icho-san
Cyperus & cluster combination	xiangsha yangwei tang	kosa-yoi-to

Cyperus & perilla formula	xiangsu san	koso-san
Cyperus, perilla & citrus formula	xingqi xiangsu san	gyoki-koso-san
D.B. & O.S. combination	longgu muli tang	ryukotu-borei-to
Dandelion combination	pugongying tang	hokoei-to
Dianthus formula	bazheng san	hachi-sei-san
Dioscorea combination	sishen tang	sisin-to
Elsholtzia combination	xiangru yin	koju-in
Elsholtzia ten combination	shiwei xiangru yin	jiumi-koju-in
Eriobotrya & ophiopogon combination	qingzao jiufei tang	seiso-kyuhai-to
Eucommia & achyranthes	weizheng fang	isho-ho
Evodia & pinellia combination	yannian banxia tang	ennen-hange-to
Evodia combination	wuzhuyu tang	gosyuyu-to
Forsythia & laminaria combination	sanzhong huijian tang	sanju-kiken-to

Forsythia & lonicera formula	zhi touchuang yi fang	zi-zuso-ippo
Forsythia & rhubarb formula	liangge san	ryokaku-san
Fritillaria & platycodon formula	ningsou wan	neiso-gan
G.L. & aconite combination with ginseng	sini jia renshen tang	sigyaku-ka-ninzin-to
G.P. & ginseng formula	ganjiang renshen banxia wan	kankyo-ninzin-to
Galanoa & chih-shih combination	liangzhi tang	ryoki-to
Gambir formula	gouteng san	tyoto-san
Gardenia & hoelen formula	wu lin san	gorin-san
Gardenia & mentha combination	qingliang yin	seiryo-yin
Gardenia & phellodendron combination	zhizi bopi tang	shisi-hekihi-to
Gardenia & vitex combination	xigan mingmu tang	senkan-meimoku-to
Gasping formula	xiangsheng podi wan	kyosei-hateki-gan

Gelatin & aristolochia combination	bufei ajiao tang	hohai-akyo-to
Gelatin & artemisia 4 combination	jiao ai siwu tang	kyogai-simotsu-to
Gentiana combination	longdan xiegan tang	ryutan-syakan-to
Ginger & hoelen combination	ling jiang shu gan tang	ryo-kyo-zyutu-kan-to
Ginseng & astragalus combination	buzhong yiqi tang	hotyu-ekki-to
Ginseng & atractylodes forrmula	shen ling baishu san	sanrei-hakuzyutu-san
Ginseng & ginger combination	renshen tang	ninzin-to
Ginseng & gypsum combination	baihu jia renshen tang	byakko-ka- ninzin-to
Ginseng & longan combination	quipi tang	kihi-to
Ginseng & mentha formula	renshen baidu san	ninzin-hadoku-san
Ginseng & perilla combination	shen su yin	zinso-in
Ginseng & tang-kuei formula	renshen dan shao san	ninzin-tosyaku-san

Ginseng & tang kuei ten combination	shihquan dabu tang	zyuzen-taiho-to
Ginseng & zanthoxylum combination	lizhong anhui tang	richu-ankai-to
Ginseng & zizyphus formula	tianwang buxin dan	teno-hosin-tan
Ginseng combination	renshen yangrong tang	ninzin-yoei-to
Ginseng longan & bupleurum combination	jiawei guipi tang	kami-kihi-to
Ginseng stomach combination	renshen yang wei tang	ninzin-yoi-to
Gleditsia combination	tuoli xiaodu yin	takuri-shodoku-in
Gypsum combination	baihu tang	byakko-to
Gypsum, coptis & scute combination	sanhuang shihgao tang	sano-sekko-to
H.A. & licorice combination	fuling xingren gancao tang	bukuryo-kyonin-kanzo-to
Hoelen & alisma combination	fenxiao tang	bunsho-to
Hoelen & areca combination	wupi yin	gohi-in

Hoelen & atractylodes combination	ling gui shu gan tang	ryo-kei-zyutu-to
Hoelen & bamboo combination	wendan tang	untan-to
Hoelen & cuscuta formula	fu tu tan	buku-to-to
Hoelen & jujube combination	jiangzhong tang	kentyu-to
Hoelen & polyporus formula	zhizhuo guben wan	chidaku-kohon-gan
Hoelen & schizandra combination	ling gan jiang wei xin xia ren tang	ryokan-kyomi-singejin-to
Hoelen combination	fuling yin	bukuryo-in
Hoelen five herbs formula	wuling san	gorei-san
Holen, atractylodes areca combination	daoshui fuling tang	dosui-bukurei-to
Hoelen, G.L. & aconite combination	fuling sini tang	bukuryo-sigyaku-to
Hoelen, licorice & jujube combination	ling gui gan zao tang	ryo-kei-kan-zo-to
Hoelen, licorice & schizandra combination	ling gui wei gan tang	reiki-mikan-to

Hoelen, magnolia & apricot formula	zhichuan fang	chisen-ho
Inula & hematite combination	xuanfuhua daizheshi tang	senpuku-kadai-syaseki-to
Kaki combination	shidi tang	shitei-to
Kaolin & limonite combination	chishizhi yuyuliang tang	shakusekishi-uyoryo-to
Kaolin & oryza combination	taohua tang	toka-to
Licorice & aconite combination	gancao fuzi tang	kanzo-fusi-to
Licorice & ginger combination	gancao ganjiang tang	kanzo-kankyo-to
Licorice & hoelen combination	fuling gancao tang	bukuryo-kanzo-to
Licorice & jujube combination	gan mai dazao tang	kanbaku-taiso-to
Licorice (baked) combination	zhigancao tang	sya-kanzo-to
Licorice, aconite & ginger pulse combination	tongmo sini tang	tsumyaku-sigyaku-to
Lily combination	baihe gujin tang	byakugo-kokin-to
Lindera & cyperus formula	zhengqi tianxiang san	shoki-tenko-san
Lindera formula	wuyao shunqi san	uyaku-junki-san

Linum & rhubarb combination	runchang tang	zyuntyo-to
Lithospermum & o.s. combination	zigen muli tang	shikon-borei-to
Lithospermum ointment	ziyun gao	siun-ko
Lonicera & forsythia formula	Yingiao san	gingyo-san
Lonicera & rehmannia formula	baidu san	haidoku-san
Lotus & citrus combination	qipi tang	keihi-to
Lotus seed combination	qingxin lianzi yin	seisin-rensi-in
Lotus stamen formula	jinsuo gujing wan	kinsa-kosei-gan
Ludwigia formula	denghua baidu san	toka-haidoku-san
Lycium formula	huanshao dan	kansho-tan
Lycium, chrysanthemum, rehmannia formula	qi ju dihuang wan	kokiku-jio-gan
M.H. & apricot seed combinatiion	ma xing gang shi tang	makyo-kanseki-to
M.H. & asarum combinatiion	mahuang fuzi xixin tang	mao-fushi-saishin-to

M.H. & cimicifuga combination	shishen tang	jishin-to
M.H. & coix combination	ma xing yi gan tang	makyo-yokukan-to
M.H. & ginko combination	dingchuan tang	teizen-to
M.H. & ginseng combination	xuming tang	zoku-mei-to
M.H. magnolia combination	shenmi tang	sinpi-to
M.H. & morus formula	huagai san	kagai-san
M.H. combination	mahuang tang	mao-to
Ma-huang & gypsum combination	yuebi tang	eppi-to
Ma-huang & peony combinaiton	xiaoxuming tang	sho-zokumei-to
Ma-huang, aconite & licorice combination	mahuang fuzi gancao tang	mao-fusi-kanzo-to
Ma-huang, gypsum & pinellia combination	yuebi jia banxia tang	eppi-ka-hange-to
Ma-huang, licorice & apricot seed combinaiton	sanao tang	sanyo-to

Magnolia & alisman combination	buqi jianzhong tang	hoki-kenchu-to
Magnolia & atractylodes combination	shipi yin	jitsuhi-in
Magnolia & ginger formula	pingwei san	heii-san
Magnolia & gypsum combination	xinyi qingfei tang	sini-seihai-to
Magnolia & hoelen combination	wei ling tang	irei-to
Magnolia & saussurea combination	houpo wenzhong tang	koboku-unchu-to
Magnolia 3 combination	houpo sanwu tang	koboku-sanbutsu-to
Magnolia 7 combination	houpo qiwu tang	koboku-shichimotsu-to
Magnolia flower formula	xinyi san	shini-san
Major blue dragon combination	daqinglong tang	dai-seiryu-to
Major bupleurum combination	da chaihu tang	dai-saiko-to
Major four herbs combination	sijunzi tang	sikunsi-to

Major rhubarb combination	da chengqi tang	dai-zyoki-to
Major siler combination	da fangfeng tang	dai-bohu-to
Major six herbs combination	liujunzi tang	rokkunsi-to
Major zanthoxylum combination	da jianzhong tang	dai-kentyu-to
Mantis formula	sangpiaoxiao-san	sohyosho-san
Minor bupleurum combination	xiao chaihu tang	syo-saiko-to
Minor cinnamon & paeonia combination	xiao jianzhong tang	syo-kentyu-to
Minor rhubarb combination	xiao chenqi tang	syo-zyoki-to
Minor trichosanthes combination	xiao xianxiong tang	syo-kankyo-to
Morus & chrysanthemumm combination	sang ju yin	so-kiku-in
Morus & lycium formula	xienbai san	sya-haku-san
Morus & platycodon formula	dunsou san	ton-so-san
Moutan persica combination	tenglong tang	to-ryu-to

Mume formula	wumei wan	ubai-gan
Musk & catechu formula	qili san	shichi-rin-san
Ophiopogon & asarum combination	qingshang juantong tang	seijo-shokutsu-to
Ophiopogon & trichosanthes combination	maimendong yinzi	bakumondo-insi
Ophiopogon combination	maimendong tang	bakumondo-to
Peony & licorice combination	shaoyao gancao tang	syakuyaku-kanzo-to
Peony combination	shaoyao tang	syakuyaku-to
Peony, licorice & aconite combination	shaoyao gancao fuzi tang	syakuyaku-kanzo-fusi-to
Perilla fruit combination	suzi jiangqi tang	soshi-koki-to
Persica & rhubarb combination	taohe chenqi tang	tokaku-zyoki-to
Phellodendron combination	ziyin jianghuo tang	ziin-koka-to
Pinellia & arisaema combination	qingshi huadan tang	seishitsu-kantan-to
Pinellia & gardenia combination	lige tang	rikaku-to

Pinellia & gastrodia combination	banxia baizhu tianma tang	hange-byakuzyutu-tenma-to
Pinellia & ginger combination	shenjiang xiexin tang	shokyo-syashin-to
Pinellia & ginseng combination	banxia liujunzi tang	hange-rokkunsi-to
Pinellia & hoelen combination	xiao banxia jia fuling tang	syo-hange-ka-bukuryo-to
Pinellia & licorice combination	gancao xiexin tang	kanzo-syasin-to
Pinellia & magnolia combination	banxia houpo tang	hange-koboku-to
Pinellia, atractylodes & agastache formula	buhuanjin zhengqi san	fukankin-shoki-to
Platycodon & chih-shih formula	painong san	haino-san
Platycodon & fritillary combination	qingfei tang	seihai-to
Platycodon & gypsum combination	jiegeng shigao tang	kikyo-sekko-to
Platycodon & jujube combination	painong tang	haino-to
Platycodon & schizone-peta formula	zhisou san	shiso-san

Platycodon combination	jiegeng tang	kikyo-to
Polyporus combination	zhuling tang	tyorei-to
Pteropus & bulrush formula	shixiao san	shissho-san
Pueraria & carthamus combination	gegen honghua tang	kakkon-koka-to
Pueraria & magnolia combination	gegen tang jia xinyi chuanxiong	kakkon-to-ka-senkyu-sini
Pueraria combination	gegen tang	kakkon-to
Pueraria flower combination	gehua jiexing tang	kakka-kaisei-to
Pueraria combination	qingbi tang	seibi-to
Pueraria, coptis & scute combination	gegen huanglian huangqin tang	kakkkon-oren-ogon-to
Rehmannia & akebia formula	daochi san	doseki-san
Rehmannia & gypsum combination	yunu jian	gyoku-nyo-sen
Rehmannia & lonicera formula	baidu san	haidoku-san

Rehmannia eight formula	bawei dehuang wan	hatimi-jio-gan
Rehmannia six formula	liuwei dehuang wan	rokumi-gan
Rhubarb & aconite combination	dahuang fuzi tang	daio-fusi-to
Rhubarb & licorice combination	dahuang gancao tang	daio-kanzo-to
Rhubarb & mirabilitum combination	diaowei chenqi tang	tyoi-zyoki-to
Rhubarb & moutan combination	dahuang mudanpi tang	daio-botanpi-to
Rhubarb combination	dahuang huanglian xiexin tang	daio-oren-syasin-to
Saussurea & cardamon combinatinon	xiangsha liujunzi tang	kosa-rok-kunsi-to
Saussurea & coptis formula	xiang lian wan	koren-gan
Schizonepeta & forsythia combination	jingjie lianqiao tang	keigai-rengyo-to
Schizonepeta & pinellia formula	jinfeicao san	kinfusso-san

Schizonepeta & siler formula	jing fang baidu san	keibo-haidoku-san
Scute & cimicifuga combination	puji xiaodu yin	fusei-syodoku-in
Scute & licorice combination	huangqin tang	ogon-to
Scute 3 herb combination	sanwu huangqin tang	sanmotu-ogon-to
Scute combination	zishen tonger tang	zizin-tsuji-to
Siler & chianghuo combination	jiawei baxian tang	kami-hassen-to
Siler & coix combination	qingshang fangfeng tang jia yiyiren	seijo-bofu-toka -yokuinin
Siler & licorice formula	xiehuang san	sya-o-san
Siler & platycodon formula	fangfeng tongsheng san	bohu-tusyo-san
Siler combination	qingshang fangfeng tang	sei-zyo-bohu-to
Smilax & akebia combination	xiangchuan jiedu ji	kosen-gedoku-zai
Stephania & astragalus combination	fangji huangqi tang	boi-ogi-to

Stephania & carthamus combination	shufeng huoxie tang	sohu-kakketsu-to
Stephania & ginseng combination	mufangji tang	moku-boi-to
Stephania & hoelen combination	fangji fuling tang	boi-bukuryo-to
Sweet combination	ganlu yin	kanro-in
Tang-kuei & anemarrhena combination	danggui niantong tang	toki-sentsu-to
Tang-kuei & arctium formula	xiaofeng san	syohu-san
Tang-kuei & atractylodes combination	lianzhu yin	ren-zyu-in
Tang-kuei & bupleurum formula	xiaoyao san	syoyo-san
Tang-kuei & carthamus combination	tongdao san	tu-do-san
Tang-kuei & cimicifuga combination	qingre buqi tang	seinetsu-hoki-to
Tang-kuei & cyperus combination	nushen san	nyosin-san

Tang-kuei & evodia combination	wenjing tang	unkei-to
Tang-kuei & gambir combination	qiwu jiangxia tang	sitimotu-koka-to
Tang-kuei & gardenia combination	wenqing yin	unsei-in
Tang-kuei & gelatin combination	xiong gui jiao ai tang	kyuki-kyogai-to
Tang-kuei & ginger combination	shenghua tang	seika-to
Tang-kuei & ginger eight combination	bazhen tang	hattin-to
Tang-kuei & jujube combination	danggui sini tang	toki-sigyaku-to
Tang-kuei & magnolia combination	wuji san	gosyaku-san
Tang-kuei & parsley combination	antai yin	an-tai-in
Tang-kuei & peony formula	danggui shaoyao san	toki-syakuyaku-san
Tang-kuei & persica combination	fuyuan huoxie tang	fukugen-kakketsu-to
Tang-kuei & pinellia combination	pinggan liuqi yin	heikan-ryuki-in

Tang-kuei & rehmannia combination	buyin tang	hoin-to
Tang-kuei & tribulus combination	danggui yinzi	toki-insi
Tang-kuei combination	qianjin danggui tang	senkin-toki-to
Tang-kuei eight herbs formula	bawei daixia fang	hachimi-taika-ho
Tang-kuei formula	dangqui san	toki-san
Tang-kuei four formula	siwu tang	simotu-to
Tang-kuei sixteen herbs combination	shiliuwei liuqi yin	jyurokumi-ryuki-in
Tang-kuei, cinnamon & peony combination	danggui jianzhong tang	toki-kentyu-to
Tang-kuei, evodia & ginger combination	danggui sini jia wuzhuyu shenjiang tang	toki-sigyaku-ka-gosyuyu-syokyo-to
Tang-kuei & astragalus combination	dangqui buxie tang	toki-hoketsu-to
Tokoro combination	bijie fenqing yin	hikai-bunsei-in
Trichosanthes & chih- shih combination	guolou zhishi tang	katsuro-kijitsu-to

Trichosanthes, bakeri & pinellia combination	gualou xiebai banxia tang	katsuro-hihaku-hange-to
Tuhuo & vaeicum combination	duhuo jisheng tang	dokukatsu-kisei-to
Vita combination	zhenwu tang	sinbu-to
W.T.T.C.	le shi shu	raku-teki-jo
Wu-tou & cinnamon combination	wutou guizhi tang	uzu-keisi-to
Xanthium formula	canger san	soji-san
Zanthoxylum combination	jieji shujiao tang	kaikyu-shokushuku-to
Zizyphus combination	suan-zao-ren-tang	sansonin-to

Appendix 3

Anti-HIV, Immunostimulating Polysaccharide-srich, and Interferon-inducing Chinese Herbs

Anti-HIV Chinese Herbs

References

1. R. Shihman Chang and H.W. Yeung, "Inhibition of Growth of Human Immunodeficiency Virus by Crude Extracts of Chinese Medicinal Herbs". Antiviral Research, 9 (1988), pages 163-176.
2. Chinese Herbs Screened for Anti-HIV Activity. AIDS Treatment News No.61, July 29, 1988, page 4-5.
3. Chinese Herbs show early result; Model for Community-based Trials ? AIDS Treatment News No. 65, Sept. 23, 1988, page 1-2.

Name	Pharmacentical Name	Pin-Yin
Arctium	Arctii Fructus	Niu-Bang-Zi
Cibotium	Cibotii Rhizoma	Gou-Ji
Coptis	Coptidis Rhizoma	Huang-Lian
Epimedium	Epimedii Herba	Yin-Yang-Huo
Licorice	Glycyrrhizae Radix	Gan-Cao
Lithospermum	Lithospermi Radix	Zi-Cao
Lonicera	Lonicerae Flos	Jin-Yin-Hua
Prunella	Prunellae Spica	Xia-Ku-Cao
Senecio	Senecionis Herba	Qian-Li-Guang
Viloa	Viloae Herba	Zi-Hua-Di-Ding

* Woodwardia and Cibotium are the same functional herb in Oriental Materia Medica.

Immunostimulating Polysaccharide-rich Chinese Herbs

References

1. Tsung, P.-K. and Hsu, H.Y. Immunology and Chinese Herbal Medicine. Oriental Healing Arts Institute,Long Beach, CA.1986
2. Tsung, P.-K. Anti-cancer and Immunostimulating Polysaccharides. OHAI Bull. 12, 1-10, 1987
3. Tsung, P.-K. Immunity, Aging and Chinese Herbs. OHAI Bull. 13, 96-100, 1988

Name	Pharmaceutical Name	Pin-Yin
Acanthopanax	Acanthopanacis Radicis Cortex	Wu-Jia-Pi
Artemisia	Artemisiae Argyi Folium	Ai-Ye
Astragalus	Astragali Radix	Huang-Qi
Codonopsis	Codonopsis Pilosulae Radix	Dang-shen
Coix	Coicis Semen	Yi-Yi-Ren
Ginseng	Ginseng Radix	Ren-Shen
Hoelen	Poria	Fu-Ling
Lithospermum	see Anti-HIV Herbs	
Oldenlandia	Oldenlandiae Herba	Bai-Hua-She-She-Cao
Omphalia	Omphalia	Lei-Wan
Polyporus	Polyporus	Zhu-Ling
Tang-Kuei	Angelicae Radix	Dang-Gui

Interferon-inducing Chinese Herbs

References

1. Kojima, Y. From the Discovery of Interferon to Chinese Medicine. The 22nd Honomi Kanpo Seminar, Nagoya 1984, p.11-38.
2. Tamamura, S., Shibukawa, N., Kojima, Y.J. Med. Pharm. Wakan-Yaku. 72-73, 1984
3. Meng, S.Y. Chin J. Integr. Med. 3, 374-375, 1983

Agkistrodon halys	Indigo pulverata levis
Angelica dahurica	Lentinus Edode
Angelica sinensis	Lonicera japonica
Atractylodes ovata	Lycium chinensis
Astragalus membranaceus	Morinda officinalis
Benincasa Cerifera	Morus alba
Camptotheca acuminata	Paeonia lactiflora
Carthamus tinclorius	Panax ginseng Meyer
Codonopsis radix	Polygonum multiflorum
Coptis chinensis	Polygonatum officinalis
Cucumis melo	Polyporus umbellatus
Curcuma zedoaria	Poria cocos
Cuscuta chinensie	Rehmannia glutinosa
Dioscorea batatas	Schizandra chinensis
Ganoderma lucidum	Scutellaria baicalensis
Glycyrrhiza uralensis	Taraxicum mongolicum

Appendix 4

Chinese Herbal Formulas Used For
Aging-Associated Diseases

1. Heart and Circulatory Diseases

For heart failure: Valvular disease, angina pectoris, myocardial infarction: Bupleurum and Dragon Bone Combination

2. Hypertension and Arteriosclerosis:

Coptis amd Rhubarb Combination

3. Kidney diseases and Urologic Disorders

For nephritis and nephrosis: Hoelen Five Herbs Formula
To treat cystitis, urethritis and prostatomegaly:
Lotus Seed Combination

4. Diabetes: Rehmannia Eight Formula

5. Rheumatoid Arthritis

Cinnamon, Atractylodes and Aconite Combination

6. Cataracts: Rehmannia Eight Formula

7. Respiratory Diseasee

For acute bronchitis: Ma-huang and Apricot Seed Combination
For chronic bronchitis and emphysema: Platycodon and Fritillaria Combination
For bronchial asthma: Minor Bupleurum Combination plus Pinellia and Magnolia Combinaiton

8. Liver Disorders

For hepatitis: Minor Bupleurum Combination
For Cholelithiasis and cholecystitis: Bupleurum and Cinnamon Combination

9. Gastrointestinal Disorders

For gastritis: Pinellia Combination
For gastric and duodenal ulcers: Pinellia Combination
For diarrhea: Pinellia Combination
For constipation: Coptis and Rhubarb Combination

10. Gynecological Disorders

For menopausal and stagnant blood disorders: Cinnamon and Hoelen Formula
For chill syndrome: Tang-Kuei and Peony Formula
For insomnia: Ginseng, Longan and Bupleurum Combination

Appendix 5

Herbal Formulas Recommended for Allergies

Bronchial Asthma
>Minor Bupleurum Combination plus Pinellia and Magnolia Combination

Chronic B-type Hepatitis
>Minor Bupleurum Combination

Dermatitis
>Bupleurum & Schizonepeta Combination

Drug Allegy
>Hoelen Five Herb Formula

Hay Fever
>Pueraria & Magnolia Combination

Allergic Rhinitis
>Minor Blue Dragon Combination

Hives
>Bupleurum & Schizonepeta Combination

Nephritis
>Bupleurum & Hoelen Combination

Thyroiditis
>Baked Licorice Combination

Tubercular Lesions(Tuberculosis)
>Ginseng & Astragalus Combination

Ulcerous Intestinitis
>Astragalus Combination

Appendix 6

The Commonly-used Marker Constituents of Herbs

Herb	Main Constituent
1. Alisma	11-Deoxyalisol C
2. Almond	Amygdalin
3. Aristolochia	Sinomenine
4. Bupleurum	Saikosaponin
5. Cinnamon	Cinnamic aldehyde
6. Citrus	Hesperidin
7. Clove	Eugenol
8. Cnidium	Ferulic acid
9. Coptis	Berberine
10. Cornus	Loganin
11. Evodia	Evodiamine
12. Gardenia	Geniposide
13. Ginger	6-Gingerol
14. Licorice	Glycyrrhizin
15. Magnolia	Magnorol
16. Ma-huang	Ephedrine
17. Mentha	Menthol
18. Moutan bark	Paeonol
19. Peony	Paeoniflorin
20. Persica	Amygdalin
21. Phellodendron	Berberine
22. Pueraria	Diadzein
23. Rhubarb	Sennoside A
24. Scute	Baicalin

For further information concerning Chinese herbal medicine, contact the following organizations:

Institute of Chinese Herb

16 Almond Tree Lane
Irvine, CA. 92715
Phone (714) 828-9316

7439 La Palma Ave. #167
Buena Park, CA 90620
Phone (714) 828-9316

Nu Life Systems

2675 W. Woodland Dr.
Anaheim, CA. 92801
Phone (714) 828-9242
FAX (714) 761-3720